# Opioid–Use Disorders
in Pregnancy

# Opioid-Use Disorders in Pregnancy

## Management Guidelines for Improving Outcomes

Edited by
**Tricia E. Wright**
University of Hawaii

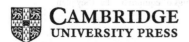

**CAMBRIDGE**
UNIVERSITY PRESS

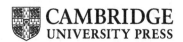

Shaftesbury Road, Cambridge CB2 8EA, United Kingdom

One Liberty Plaza, 20th Floor, New York, NY 10006, USA

477 Williamstown Road, Port Melbourne, VIC 3207, Australia

314–321, 3rd Floor, Plot 3, Splendor Forum, Jasola District Centre, New Delhi – 110025, India

103 Penang Road, #05–06/07, Visioncrest Commercial, Singapore 238467

Cambridge University Press is part of Cambridge University Press & Assessment,
a department of the University of Cambridge.

We share the University's mission to contribute to society through the pursuit of
education, learning and research at the highest international levels of excellence.

www.cambridge.org
Information on this title: www.cambridge.org/9781108400985

DOI: 10.1017/9781108231695

First published 2018

*A catalogue record for this publication is available from the British Library*

*Library of Congress Cataloging-in-Publication data*
Names: Wright, Tricia E., editor.
Title: Opioid-use disorders in pregnancy: management guidelines for improving outcomes /
    edited by Tricia E. Wright.
Description: New York, NY : Cambridge University Press, 2018. | Includes bibliographical
    references and index.
Identifiers: LCCN 2018008862 | ISBN 9781108400985 (pbk.)
Subjects: | MESH: Opioid-Related Disorders—therapy | Pregnant Women | Prenatal Care |
    Postnatal Care | Pregnancy
Classification: LCC RG580.S75 | NLM WM 284 | DDC 618.3/686—dc23 LC record
    available at https://lccn.loc.gov/2018008862

ISBN    978-1-108-40098-5    Paperback

# Contents

# Contributors

**Soraya Asadi, MD, FASAM**
Assistant Professor, Psychiatry, Loyola
University Stritch School of Medicine; Medical
Director, Opioid Treatment Program, Hines
Veterans Administration Hospital

**Margaret S. Chisolm, MD**
Associate Professor and Vice Chair for Education
Psychiatry & Behavioral Sciences, Johns
Hopkins University School of Medicine

**Carl Christensen, FACOG, DFASAM**
Associate Clinical Professor, Wayne State University;
Medical Director, Christensen Recovery Services

**Loretta Finnegan, MD**
Executive Officer, The College on Problems of Drug
Dependence, Inc., Finnegan Consulting, LLC

**Alexis S. Hammond, MD, PhD**
Behavioral Pharmacology Research Unit,
Department of Psychiatry and Behavioral Sciences,
Johns Hopkins University School of Medicine

**Lauren M. Jansson, MD**
Associate Professor of Pediatrics, Johns
Hopkins University School of Medicine

**Hendrée E. Jones, PhD**
Executive Director, UNC Horizons; Professor,
Department of Obstetrics and Gynecology, School
of Medicine, University of North Carolina

**Karol Kaltenbach, PhD**
Director, Maternal Addiction Treatment
Education & Research (MATER);
Emeritus Professor of Pediatrics
Sidney Kimmel Medical College at
Thomas Jefferson University

**Kaylin A. Klie, MD, MA, FASAM**
Assistant Professor, Department of Family
Medicine, Denver Health, University
of Colorado School of Medicine

**Elizabeth E. Krans, MD, MSc**
Assistant Professor, Department of Obstetrics,
Gynecology and Reproductive Sciences, University
of Pittsburgh Magee–Womens Research Institute

**Lawrence Leeman, MD**
Professor, Family Medicine, University
of New Mexico School of Medicine

**Marjorie Meyer, MD, FACOG**
Associate Professor, University of
Vermont School of Medicine

**Lauren Owens, MD, MPH**
University of Washington School of Medicine

**Stephen W. Patrick, MD, MPH, MS**
Assistant Professor of Pediatrics and Health
Policy, Division of Neonatology, Vanderbilt
University School of Medicine

**Charles W. Schauberger, MD, MS, FACOG**
Gunderson Lutheran Medical Center

**Richard G. Soper, MD, JD, MS, DFASAM**
Chief Medical Officer, Center for Behavioral Wellness

**Mishka Terplan, MD, MPH, FACOG, FASAM**
Professor of Obstetrics and Gynecology and
Psychiatry, Virginia Commonwealth University

**Sebastian T. Tong, MD, MPH**
Assistant Professor of Family Medicine
and Population Health, Virginia
Commonwealth University

**Jacquelyn Starer, MD, FACOG, DFASAM**
Brigham and Women's Faulkner Hospital,
Addiction Recovery Program

**Tricia E. Wright, MD, MS, FACOG, FASAM**
Associate Professor, Obstetrics, Gynecology
and Women's Health, University of Hawaii,
John A. Burns School of Medicine

# Preface and Acknowledgments

It should come as no surprise to the reader that opioid use, misuse, addiction, and overdose deaths have reached epidemic proportions in the United States and Canada. The loss of celebrities, for example, Phillip Seymour Hoffman, Cory Montieth, Anna Nichole Smith, and Prince, to opioid overdose points out that no one is immune to the ravages of addiction. Women of childbearing age have been overrepresented in this epidemic for many reasons, which will be addressed in Chapter 1, and thus there has been an epidemic of newborn infants being treated for neonatal abstinence syndrome (NAS), also known as neonatal opioid withdrawal syndrome (NOWS). Treatment of NAS is expensive and time-consuming, which has led to ill-conceived interventions for its prevention, including incarceration of pregnant women and medically assisted withdrawal without the necessary resources to adequately treat the medical problem of addiction. Most of these interventions do not consider the whole maternal–infant dyad and the natural history of opioid-use disorders, which could lead to disastrous consequences for mothers and their families.

Those of us who specialize in the treatment of pregnant women with substance use disorders are often asked to provide best practices for the treatment of opioid-dependent pregnant women and their infants. For this reason, the idea for this book arose.

I am grateful to my coauthors, who are all experts in this field, for helping this book come to fruition and to Cambridge University Press for realizing the need for such a volume.

I would like to thank my several mentors, including but certainly not limited to William F. Haning III, Kevin Kunz, Luis B. Curet, and the late Gary Helmbrecht, who have helped me become a caring competent addiction provider for pregnant women; my chairs, Kenneth Ward, Lynnae Sauvage, and Ivica Zalud, who have always provided unquestioned support for an Ob/Gyn interested in Addiction Medicine; my colleagues in Ob/Gyn who have covered for me and cared for my patients while I lobbied for funds, traveled to speak and teach, and wrote this book; the Women's Caucus of Hawaii State Legislators, especially Suzanne Chun Oakland and Marilyn Lee, who saw the need for the clinic and provided funds for its inception; the clinic staff and especially the managers, Renee Schuetter and Jacqueline Tellei; and all the numerous women and children we have cared for who have taught me so much about strength and resilience in the face of so much adversity.

I thank the contributors to this book, who are all experts in the field. I think we have put together an amazing work and I couldn't have done it without all your efforts.

# The Opioid Epidemic and Pregnant Women

Tricia E. Wright

## The History of the Current Opioid Epidemic

Sam Quinones's *Dreamland* [1] details the current opioid epidemic and is an excellent read. Since the early 1990s, opioid use in the United States and Canada has increased more than fivefold, starting with the release of Oxycontin® by Purdue Pharmaceuticals in 1996. A half page communication by Porter and Jick [2] in *The New England Journal of Medicine* showed that among *hospitalized patients* (emphasis mine) treated with opioids, less than 1 percent developed addiction. Using this study, Purdue Pharmaceuticals marketed this new extended-release opioid to primary-care physicians as the Holy Grail for the treatment of chronic pain, a safe, non-addictive opioid. Doctors were urged and incentivized to prescribe this new wonder drug, but not trained in its safe use, leaving many of their patients vulnerable to developing addictive behaviors and resulting in death due to overdose. Later studies showed that approximately 35 percent of people treated with opioids for chronic pain go on to develop an opioid-use disorder [3]. In addition, for-profit pill mills were opened in many localities, where a patient could get a month's worth of potent opioids with a minimal history of pain and cursory exam. In addition, there was no oversight of these clinics or the patients, and patients could and frequently would frequent more than one "pain clinic," leading to huge numbers of "legal" opioids circulating around communities which had been devastated by the loss of manufacturing jobs.

Simultaneously, the American (National) Pain Society first suggested that pain be treated as the fifth vital sign, and the Joint Commission for Accreditation of Hospital Organizations (JACHO) put forth hospitals that executed this as an example of good patient care [4]. Hospital satisfaction scores have been partially based on whether or not a patient's pain was treated "adequately." This led to hospitals and emergency rooms dispensing increasing numbers of opioids, especially to white patients [5] and surgeons prescribing prolonged courses of opioids, even though the majority of patients require opioids for only three days after discharge from the hospital.

By 2010, doctors prescribed sufficient opioid(s) so that "every person in the United States could be medicated around the clock for a month" (Figure 1.1) [6]. Unlike previous opioid epidemics involving heroin, this epidemic targeted mostly white and middle class people, with many of them being women of childbearing age. Women were more likely to be prescribed opioids for pain relief than men; indeed, during the 1800s, the majority of people with opium-use disorders were women who were prescribed opium for pain relief by their physicians [7]. Physicians also prescribed higher doses of opioids and for longer periods, leading to higher overdose death rates among women [6]. Women are most likely prescribed opioids for migraine, fibromyalgia, and osteoarthritis, i.e., for all

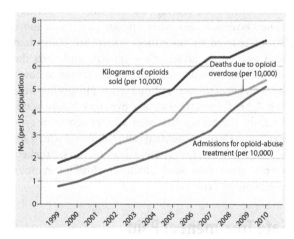

**Figure 1.1** Rates* of opioid pain reliever (OPR) overdose death, OPR treatment admissions, and kilograms of OPR sold in the United States, 1999–2010 [1]

*Age-adjusted rates per 100,000 population for OPR deaths, crude rates per 10,000 population for OPR abuse treatment admissions, and crude rates per 10,000 population for kilograms of OPR sold.

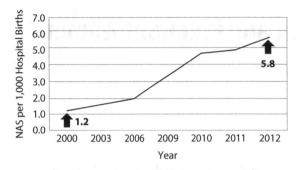

**Figure 1.2** Incidence of neonatal abstinence syndrome per 1,000 hospital births in the United States, 2000–12 [2]

conditions for which they are not effective. The great majority of women who received prescription opioids were of childbearing age, which leads to our current epidemic of infants needing treatment for neonatal abstinence syndrome (NAS) (Figure 1.2).

At the same time that the prescription opioid use epidemic came to the attention of public health officials and other authorities, another opioid was reemerging as a threat. Potent black tar heroin was smuggled from Mexico and delivered like pizza by small cells in several major cities and small towns that had never seen heroin before. This black tar, so named because it was the unrefined sticky substance directly extracted from the poppy plants, was several times more potent than the powdered heroin previously sold by dealers in big East Coast cities and was also cheap. An addict could satisfy their cravings for less than $20 per day, while Oxycontin and other opioids cost much more (if not covered by insurance). Once the pump had been primed by prescription opioids, and then the well ran dry as insurance companies refused to cover the extended-release options and pill mills were closed, heroin was there to take over this deadly trend. Recently, the heroin has been adulterated with synthetic opioids such as fentanyl and sufentanil which are hundreds of times more potent, leading to a skyrocketing rate of overdose deaths, including Phillip Seymour Hoffman and Prince.

## Safe Treatment of Pain

Opioids still have a place in the treatment of pain, though the treatment of chronic non-cancer pain with opioids is controversial. There are several safeguards that need to be used for anyone using opioids for the treatment of pain. The CDC published these guidelines

in May 2016 [8]. They include the use of prescription drug monitoring systems (PDMPs), which 49 states have implemented, and some states mandate their use by physicians before the prescription of controlled substances. Urine drug monitoring is recommended to confirm that the patient is taking the medication that is prescribed and not taking other illicit or licit substances (such as benzodiazepines) that increase the risk of overdose death. Prescribers are encouraged not to prescribe opioid for more than 3 days for acute pain, and while treating chronic pain, caution must be exercised when prescribing above 50 MME (morphine milligram equivalents) and not to exceed 90 MME [8].

There are limitations to these guidelines, and given that 35 percent of individuals treated with opioids for chronic pain will develop an opioid-use disorder, practitioners are advised to treat with care while using opioids. Ideally, the treatment of chronic pain should occur in specialized multidisciplinary pain clinics with the use of multimodal treatment options, including nonopioid medications, physical therapy, chiropractic care, psychological treatments, pain blocks, and acupuncture, as well as someone specialized in the treatment of addiction. Unfortunately, insurance coverage for such comprehensive pain clinics is inadequate, and thus there is a nationwide shortage.

## Pregnant Women and Pain

There are unfortunately few nonopioid medications that are safe in pregnancy. In addition, pregnancy increases stress on the musculoskeletal system, which can increase low back pain and other pain syndromes. Pregnancy intention should be discussed with all women being treated for chronic pain and attempts to control pain without opioids should be maximized before pregnancy. Weaning of opioids during pregnancy will be addressed in subsequent chapters, but it is important that women should not be abruptly withdrawn from opioids, as this can increase the risk of intrauterine fetal death (stillbirth), abruption, and preterm birth. All providers treating pregnant women with opioid-use disorders reported seeing an all-too-common phenomenon among women being treated at pain clinics; the prescriber, who has been managing the woman with opioids, will stop prescribing upon learning of the pregnancy, as if that will insure that the fetus is not exposed. This is a poor clinical practice, bordering on malpractice. With adequate counseling of NAS risks, many women can safely be continued on opioids during pregnancy, especially if there are no better options for treatment. Focus on nonmedication treatment of pain should be optimized (e.g., physical therapy, massage, acupuncture, and psychologic counseling such as cognitive-behavioral therapy). Unfortunately, insurance coverage for such adjunctive therapies are lacking, limiting its effectiveness in disadvantaged women (who are more vulnerable to chronic pain). Family planning will be addressed in Chapter 13, but it is of paramount importance to the optimal treatment of women with pain and with opioid-use disorders.

## Pain and Addiction: Common Threads

The vulnerability of women treated with opioids to developing an opioid-use disorder stems from many factors, including genetic vulnerability, exposure to early childhood adverse events, poverty, physical trauma, and interpersonal violence.

The American Society of Addiction Medicine (ASAM) defines addiction as a primary, chronic disease of brain reward, motivation, memory, and related circuitry. Addiction is characterized by inability to consistently abstain, impairment in behavioral control, craving, diminished recognition of significant problems with one's behaviors, and interpersonal relationships, and a dysfunctional emotional response [9]. Vulnerability to addiction is thought to be multifactorial, comprising a complex interplay of genetic and environmental causes (Figure 1.3).

Twin studies have demonstrated that genetic vulnerability comprises about 60 percent of an individual's risk of developing a substance use disorder. Interestingly studies looking at possible genetic causes of both opioid addiction and vulnerability to chronic pain have found several genes in common [10, 11]. One of these gene targets, the *COMT* gene, which regulates the metabolism of catecholamines, was found to be associated with opioid-use disorder (OUD) only in women [11]. Target gene studies comparing dependent vs. nondependent opioid users found a polymorphism in the delta opioid receptor gene *OPRD1* associated with dependent opioid use [12]. Activation of this receptor decreases persistent pain and reduces negative emotional states [13]; thus this could be a compelling target for drug development studies. Other genetic factors include polymorphisms in ADRB2 that are associated with resilience to post-traumatic stress after trauma [14], which we will see in Chapter 5 as a major factor in the development of substance use disorders.

The relationship between exposure to adverse childhood events (ACE) and substance use was first reported in 1998 [15]. Since then other studies have looked at the role of poverty [16], sexual abuse [17], and interpersonal violence [18]. All of these factors contribute to higher rates of opioid-use disorders. As we'll see in Chapters 5 and 6, trauma and interpersonal violence remain two of the greatest risk factors for the development of opioid- and other substance use disorders. These factors are also determinants of chronic pain [19–21]. Women with substance use disorders and chronic pain suffer from multiple social and health disparities and thus these disparities need to be addressed if we are to help these women, their families, and their communities recover.

## Traditional Approaches to Substance Use in Pregnancy

Focus on the risk of substance use solely on the fetus, lack of understanding of the role of the maternal-fetal dyad, and misunderstanding of the disease model of addiction have led to several public policy approaches to pregnant women with substance use disorders that have proven to be disastrous to public health as well as individual women and their families. Most of the public policy focus has been on the largely overstated and unproven risks of illicit drugs, while ignoring the real and well-known risk of the licit substances, such as alcohol and tobacco. These policies serve to prevent women from getting the prenatal care and addiction

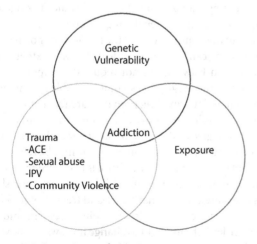

**Figure 1.3** Determinants of addiction

treatment they need and that has been shown to improve pregnancy outcomes and ameliorate the effects of the drugs.

# Traditional Approach 1: Take Away Her Children: Women with Substance Use Disorders are Unfit to Parent

There is a pervasive notion in our society that women who use illicit drugs are unfit to parent children. This is reflected in policies where children under threatened harm are removed from the home even if no child abuse or neglect is proven. Threatened harm can include a positive drug test at delivery or at any time during her prenatal course. Women with a single, positive, drug urine test have been subject to child welfare involvement and infant removal, even if confirmatory drug testing was not done, and even if she was not aware of the pregnancy at the time of her drug use. This involvement serves to place the perceived needs of the fetus above those of the pregnant woman, ignoring the rights of the pregnant woman, and the role her health plays on that of the developing fetus. It also puts the prenatal care provider into an adversarial role with the pregnant woman, as drug testing is often done without the consent or even knowledge of the pregnant woman. Instead of talking to the woman about her drug use, her social situation and other factors that can affect her and her family's health, and provided with necessary medical care (which includes addiction treatment), she is subject to unlawful search and subsequent infant abduction, which serves to perpetuate the inter-generational cycle of trauma. Women who have children removed from them, even temporarily, are more likely to get pregnant again [22]. As one mother eloquently said "I have a hole in my heart from missing those 2 months with my son. I want to go have another baby just to fill it." This can be one reason women with substance use disorders have more pregnancies and live births.

Perhaps this approach could be justified if it were shown to be effective in protecting the fetus and child from the effects of maternal drug use, but this is not the case. Policies that stress child welfare involvement actually worsen pregnancy outcomes, in that they serve as a large barrier to women obtaining prenatal care [23], which has been shown to ameliorate the effects of the substances and normalize pregnancy outcomes [24]. A single drug test does not predict parenting ability [25];

Susan Boyd found no differences between women who use drugs and those who do not in their childrearing practices [26]. In addition, in 1976, as Michael Wald said [27], "Removing a child from his family may cause serious psychological damage – damage more serious than the harm intervention was supposed to prevent."

Keeping children with the mother while she undergoes drug treatment improves the outcomes of the entire family [28]. Since the early 1990s, this model of comprehensive care has been supported by the Substance Abuse and Mental Health Services Administration's (SAMHSA) Center for Substance Abuse Treatment (CSAT), and has demonstrated success in many states [29]. Despite the success of this approach, funding was drastically cut to this program and these facilities are still available in less than half of states.

On a practical note to providers who care for women with substance use disorders, current state laws are influenced by the Child Abuse Prevention and Treatment Act (CAPTA), which was originally enacted in 1974 and most recently updated and reauthorized in 2010. The purpose of this act is to provide funding to states for child welfare services. A new CAPTA state grant eligibility requirement modifies earlier CAPTA language that mandates identifying and making "appropriate referrals" by healthcare providers to CPS – and developing service "plans for safe care" of the child – of newborns affected by prenatal drug exposure. Various states have interpreted these requirements in various ways, both in reporting requirements and what is meant by newborns affected by prenatal drug exposure. The most recent requirements also include infants affected by NAS and fetal alcohol syndrome (FAS). Knowledge of your own state laws is imperative while taking care of women with substance use disorders. Counseling women during the course of prenatal care as to the requirements of the law and your own role in reporting can help allay her fears to some extent. For example, in Hawai'i, I'm not required to report drug use during the pregnancy, so that I am able to reassure the woman I'm providing prenatal care for that I won't report her unless there are other concerns about child abuse or neglect. I do explain that if her child has NAS or if the pediatrician has concerns, she may be referred, but that the purpose of the referral is to ensure access to resources, not to remove the child from custody if she has been attending prenatal care and treatment for her substance use disorder. Providers in states with more punitive laws should fight to change the laws and advocate for your patient's rights.

## Traditional Approach 2: Lock Her Up: Incarcerated Women won't Use and Babies will be Born Healthy

This approach began in the 1980s in response to the crack cocaine epidemic and the media coverage which promised a lost generation of crack-exposed children. Despite little evidence of long-term harm in carefully controlled studies, legislators began crafting bills that would criminalize drug use during pregnancy. Strong opposition by medical societies and public health groups prevented the worst of these bills from passing [25]. To date, only one state (Tennessee) explicitly criminalized drug use during pregnancy. Given strong opposition from the American Medical Association (AMA), the American Congress of Obstetricians and Gynecologists (ACOG), the American Academy of Pediatrics (AAP), the ASAM, as well as state health and law enforcement agencies, this law was allowed to sunset in 2016. However, currently three states (Minnesota, South Dakota, and Wisconsin) consider drug use during pregnancy grounds for civil commitment and 17 states currently consider drug use during pregnancy to be child abuse [30]. States have used these statutes and others to incarcerate pregnant women who use drugs. Paltrow and Flavin [31] found 348 cases from 1973 to 2005 where women were arrested solely for using drugs during pregnancy. They have found an additional 380 cases since 2005 [30].

Problems with these policies are multitude. Incarcerated women suffer from stress, poor diet, interpersonal violence, trauma from family separation, lack of access to psychiatric, addiction and medical care, including medically assisted treatment, as well as continued access to drugs of abuse, all of which increase pregnancy complications and poor infant outcomes. These policies ignore the risks of legal drugs, including tobacco and alcohol, whose effects in many studies have shown to be more harmful than those of illicit drugs. As we saw with child abuse policies, fear of legal involvement prevents women from obtaining prenatal care and worsens outcomes. In 1997, Cornelia Whitner was 1 of 42 women systematically arrested by South Carolina police for using crack cocaine during pregnancy. She was tested at the Medical University of South Carolina without her knowledge or consent. Her conviction was upheld by the State Supreme Court, deviating from other state courts. After her conviction, admission to drug treatment decreased by 80 percent,

there was an increase in infant mortality, and a 20 percent increase in abandoned babies [32].

In addition, laws that punish pregnant women have been disproportionately directed toward women of color and women in poverty. Of the 42 women arrested under South Carolina law, 41 were African American. In addition, they only tested indigent women, not women using private insurance. Of the 384 women initially reported by Paltrow and Flavin, 59 percent were women of color [31].In a recent study looking at opioid withdrawal in pregnancy [33], there was one arm of women who were incarcerated and thus forced into withdrawal without medical assistance. About 20 percent of that group was African American compared to 4 percent African American women in the other practice settings.

I would encourage any provider in states with laws encouraging incarceration to work with their state legislators to change the laws. Providers need to advocate for their patients using an evidence-based approach.

## Traditional Approach 3: Compel Her to Get Treatment (Either through the Child Welfare or Criminal Justice System)

This approach seems the most humane on the surface, and many localities have affected this method. It is not without its problems, however, as was seen earlier, many states and localities are overwhelmed by the current epidemic and lack the resources for treatment, especially in rural areas which have been the hardest hit [34]. In Tennessee, for example, the law making it a crime to use drugs during pregnancy allowed a "safe harbor" for women who obtained drug treatment. At that time, there were only 50 residential treatment beds for pregnant women in a state with a need over 20 times that high. Good quality care is imperative for pregnant women. Treatment centers work best if they provide co-located prenatal care, women-specific, trauma-informed treatment, childcare, and transportation. These centers are rare and only present in approximately 18 states at the time of this writing.

Mandating a particular form of treatment can be problematic. In many instances, it is not the woman and her treatment provider making the treatment modality choice using shared decision making and evidence-based criteria, but an inexperienced child welfare worker or family court judge making that decision. This has led to many instances where the woman is forced off medically assisted treatment in order to maintain custody or stay out of jail. This leads to relapse and treatment failure. Relapse can be life-threatening, especially if it happens after a prolonged period of abstinence. The United States leads the developed world in maternal mortality. In at least two states that have looked at causes of maternal mortality (Maryland [35] and Colorado [36]), the leading cause is overdose in the postpartum period, so a suboptimal response to the opioid epidemic could be fueling our high maternal mortality rates.

## A Note about Language and Stigma

We have tried throughout the book to focus on *DSM-V* definitions of substance use disorder, and tried to avoid terms such as substance abuse, abuser, addict, or alcoholic.

While it may seem trivial to focus on language, it is not just "semantics" or "political correctness." There are two separate, but related, issues here, Person-first language and pejorative language. There has been an awakening in medical education to use person-first language. Person-first means that the focus should be on the person with the disease first, not the disease itself, reinforcing that people are not defined by the disease. For example, the term should be a person with diabetes, not a diabetic. By focusing on the disease and not the patient, it serves to dehumanize those suffering. This is especially evident in the addiction field. Kelly and Westerhoff [37] performed a study in 2010 with doctorate-level addiction and mental health providers who were provided with case scenarios of patients with legal difficulties from their substance use. Half the scenarios used "substance abusers" and half used "with a substance use disorder." The scenarios with substance abusers were significantly more likely to be judged as deserving punishment than the exact same scenarios as those having a substance use disorder.

Pejorative language subtly influences how people view people with diseases [38], and again serves to dehumanize those suffering and facilitates thinking of them as other or less worthy of care. Avoiding pejorative language is especially important when dealing with stigmatizing conditions. Drug and alcohol-use disorders are the most stigmatized medical conditions. When talking about pregnant women with substance use disorders, the stigma is increased by magnitudes. Terms such as "crack baby," "meth baby," and "opioids tiniest victims," serve to reinforce the belief that women

chose this disease and chose to do this to their children. This stigma serves to prevent women from getting the care they need and deserve, and influences policy makers to enact the laws we saw above which are so harmful and counterproductive. The commonly used term "babies born addicted to drugs" is completely fallacious. As said above, addiction is a disease of impaired control. Newborn infants by definition cannot be born addicted. They suffer from opioid withdrawal, which is a treatable medical condition.

## Summary

The above introduction to the genetic and social determinants of addiction was meant to enlighten the reader that no woman would willingly chose using substances during pregnancy for herself and her infant. Addiction is a chronic, relapsing, treatable medical condition which can cause complications of pregnancy if not managed, just like diabetes, high blood pressure, or lupus. With appropriate treatment, complications can be avoided, infants can be treated, and families can be preserved.

## References

1. Quinones S. *Dreamland*. New York, NY: Bloomsbury Press; 2015.

2. Porter J., Jick H. Addiction rare in patients treated with narcotics. *The New England Journal of Medicine*. 1980;302(2):123.

3. Boscarino J. A., Rukstalis M. R., Hoffman S. N., et al. Prevalence of prescription opioid-use disorder among chronic pain patients: comparison of the DSM-5 vs. DSM-4 diagnostic criteria. *Journal of Addictive Diseases*. 2011;30(3):185–94.

4. Berry P. H., Dahl J. L. The new JCAHO pain standards: implications for pain management nurses. *Pain Management Nursing: Official Journal of the American Society of Pain Management Nurses*. 2000;1(1):3–12.

5. Pletcher M. J., Kertesz S. G., Kohn M. A., Gonzales R. Trends in opioid prescribing by race/ethnicity for patients seeking care in US emergency departments. *Journal of the American Medical Association*. 2008;299(1):70–8.

6. Mack K., Jones C., Paulozzi L. *Vital Signs: Overdoses of Prescription Opioid Pain Relievers and Other Drugs Among Women – United States, 1999–2010*. 2013. Available at: www.cdc.gov/mmwr/preview/ mmwrhtml/mm6226a3.htm. Accessed June 27, 2017.

7. Kandall S. R. *Substance and Shadow: Women and Addiction in the United States*. Cambridge, MA: Harvard University Press; 1999.

8.  Dowell D. H. T., Chou R. CDC guideline for prescribing opioids for chronic pain – United States, 2016. *MMWR Recommendations and Reports.* 2016;65(1):1–49. DOI: http://dx.doi.org/10.15585/mmwr.rr6501e1.

9.  American Society of Addiction Medicine. Available at: www.asam.org/quality-practice/definition-of-addiction. Accessed June 27, 2017.

10. Trescot A. M., Faynboym S. A review of the role of genetic testing in pain medicine. *Pain Physician.* 2014;17(5):425–45.

11. Reed B., Butelman E. R., Yuferov V., Randesi M., Kreek M. J. Genetics of opiate addiction. *Current Psychiatry Reports.* 2014;16(11):504.

12. Randesi M., van den Brink W., Levran O., et al. Variants of opioid system genes are associated with non-dependent opioid use and heroin dependence. *Drug and Alcohol Dependence.* 2016;168:164–9.

13. Pradhan A. A., Befort K., Nozaki C., Gaveriaux-Ruff C., Kieffer B. L. The delta opioid receptor: an evolving target for the treatment of brain disorders. *Trends in Pharmacological Sciences.* 2011;32(10):581–90.

14. Liberzon I., King A. P., Ressler K. J., et al. Interaction of the ADRB2 gene polymorphism with childhood trauma in predicting adult symptoms of posttraumatic stress disorder. *JAMA Psychiatry.* 2014;71(10):1174–82.

15. Felitti V. J., Anda R. F., Nordenberg D., et al. Relationship of childhood abuse and household dysfunction to many of the leading causes of death in adults. The adverse childhood experiences (ACE) study. *American Journal of Preventive Medicine.* 1998;14(4):245–58.

16. Cohen S., Janicki-Deverts D., Chen E., Matthews K. A. Childhood socioeconomic status and adult health. *Annals of the New York Academy of Sciences.* 2010;1186:37–55.

17. Draucker C. B., Mazurczyk J. Relationships between childhood sexual abuse and substance use and sexual risk behaviors during adolescence: An integrative review. *Nursing Outlook.* 2013;61(5):291–310.

18. Stewart D. E., Vigod S., Riazantseva E. New developments in intimate partner violence and management of its mental health sequelae. *Current Psychiatry Reports.* 2016;18(1):4.

19. Ford-Gilboe M., Varcoe C., Noh M., et al. Patterns and predictors of service use among women who have separated from an abusive partner. *Journal of Family Violence.* 2015;30(4):419–31.

20. Spiegel D. R., Chatterjee A., McCroskey A. L., et al. A review of select centralized pain syndromes: relationship with childhood sexual abuse, opiate prescribing, and treatment implications for the primary care physician. *Health Services Research and Managerial Epidemiology.* 2015;2:2333392814567920.

21. Newman A. K., Van Dyke B. P., Torres C. A., et al. The relationship of sociodemographic and psychological variables to chronic pain variables in a low-income population. *Pain.* 2017;158(9):1687–96.

22. Wright T. E., Schuetter R., Fombonne E., Stephenson J., Haning W. F., 3rd. Implementation and evaluation of a harm-reduction model for clinical care of substance using pregnant women. *Harm Reduction Journal.* 2012;9(1):5.

23. Roberts S., Pies C. Complex calculations: how drug use during pregnancy becomes a barrier to prenatal care. *Maternal and Child Health Journal.* 2011;15(3):333–41.

24. El-Mohandes A., Herman A. A., Nabil El-Khorazaty M., et al. Prenatal care reduces the impact of illicit drug use on perinatal outcomes. *Journal of Perinatology: Official Journal of the California Perinatal Association.* 2003;23(5):354–60.

25. Paltrow L. M. Governmental responses to pregnant women who use alcohol or other drugs. *DePaul Journal of Health Care Law* 2005;8(2):461. Available at: http://via.library.depaul.edu/jhcl/vol8/iss2/7.

26. Boyd S. C. *Mothers and Illicit Drugs: Transcending the Myths.* Toronto, ON: University of Toronto Press; 1999.

27. Wald M. S. State intervention on behalf of 'neglected' children: a search for realistic standards. *Stanford Law Review.* 1976;28:623–706.

28. Jackson V. Residential treatment for parents and their children: the Village experience. *Science and Practice Perspectives.* 2004;2(2):44–53.

29. SAMHSA, Center for Substance Abuse Treatment (CSAT). Telling their stories: reflections of the 11 original grantees that piloted residential treatment for women and children for CSAT. *NCJRS.* 2001;46. Available at: www.ncjrs.gov/App/Publications/abstract.aspx?ID=196576. Accessed June 27, 2017.

30. Stone R. Pregnant women and substance use: fear, stigma, and barriers to care. *Health & Justice.* 2015;3(2).

31. Paltrow L., Flavin J. Arrests of and forced interventions on pregnant women in the United States, 1973–2005: implications for women's legal status and public health. *Journal of Health Politics, Policy and Law.* April 2013;38(2). DOI: http://dx.doi.org/10.1215/03616878-1966324.

32. Paltrow L., Cohen D., Carey C. Overview: governmental responses to pregnant women who use alcohol or other drugs. *Women's Law Project and the National Advocates for Pregnant Women.* 2000. Available at: www.csdp.org/news/news/gov_response_review.pdf. Accessed June 27, 2017.

33. Bell J., Towers C. V., Hennessy M. D., et al. Detoxification from opiate drugs during pregnancy.

*American Journal of Obstetrics and Gynecology.* 2016;215(3):374.e1–6.

34. Terplan M., Longinaker N., Appel L. Women-centered drug treatment services and need in the United States, 2002–2009. *American Journal of Public Health.* 2015;105(11):e50–4.

35. Maryland Department of Health and Mental Hygiene Prevention and Health Promotion Administration. Maryland Maternal Mortality Review: 2015 Annual Report.

36. Metz T. D., Rovner P., Hoffman M. C., et al. Maternal deaths from suicide and overdose in Colorado,

2004–2012. *Obstetrics and Gynecology.* 2016;128(6):1233–40.

37. Kelly J. F., Westerhoff C. M. Does it matter how we refer to individuals with substance-related conditions? A randomized study of two commonly used terms. *The International Journal on Drug Policy.* 2010;21(3):202–7.

38. Kelly J. F., Saitz R., Wakeman S. Language, substance use disorders, and policy: the need to reach consensus on an "addiction-ary". *Alcoholism Treatment Quarterly.* 2016;34(1):116–23.

# 2

# Screening, Brief Intervention and Referral to Treatment for Opioid Use Disorders in Pregnancy

Tricia E. Wright

Substance use is common in women of childbearing age. Prior to pregnancy, approximately 55 percent of women drink alcoholic beverages, 23 percent smoke cigarettes, and 10 percent use either illicit drugs or prescription drugs without a prescription [1]. Although most women are able to quit or cut back harmful substances during pregnancy, many are unwilling or unable to stop. National survey data indicate that during pregnancy, 10 percent of women drink alcohol (4 percent binge, i.e. have 5 or more alcoholic drinks on the same occasion on at least 1 day in the past 30 days), 15 percent smoke cigarettes [1], and 5 percent use an illicit substance. This makes substance use as more common than many conditions routinely screened for and assessed during prenatal care (PNC), such as cystic fibrosis, gestational diabetes, anemia, postpartum depression, or preeclampsia. Moreover, substance use during pregnancy is both costly and harmful. Substance use during pregnancy is associated with poor pregnancy outcomes, including preterm birth, low-birth weight, birth defects, developmental delays, and miscarriage [2]. Long-term effects on the mother and infant include medical, legal, familial and social problems, some of which are lifelong and costly [3, 4].

The perinatal provider, therefore, has an important medical and ethical role in screening for substance use, counseling women on the importance of avoiding harmful substances, supporting their behavioral change, and referring women with addiction to specialized treatment when needed [5, 6]. This process, known as SBIRT (screening, brief intervention, and referral to treatment), represents a public health approach to the delivery of early intervention and treatment services for persons with substance use disorders (SUDs) [7] (Figure 2.1). Its use in emergency, general primary care, and obstetric settings for alcohol and tobacco has been recommended by the U.S. Preventive Services Task Force [8, 9] as well as by professional societies such as the American College of Obstetricians and Gynecologists (ACOG) [10].

Unfortunately, a number of barriers have limited SBIRT's public health impact, particularly during pregnancy. First, although universal screening for substance use is recommended during pregnancy [11], many women are not screened [12] or not screened with evidence-based screening tools [13]. Providers often feel overwhelmed by the number of disease states for which they are expected to screen and/or feel inadequately trained to screen for substance use [14]. Clinicians may also question the clinical utility of screening and the likelihood that women will reduce substance use or attain abstinence; conversely, they may be under the impression that they do not have patients who use substances in their practices or may not want to "play police" due to mandatory reporting requirements in some states [15]. In addition, providers may feel at a loss of what to do if they encounter a patient with a SUD or unsure how to help the patient if unaware of community resources for treatment. Finally, inadequate reimbursement for evaluation and management services is a disincentive to provide preventative care even in the case of pregnant women [16].

Second, failure to disclose substance use (or incomplete disclosure) is also common, and further complicates efforts to identify at-risk women [17–21]. Pregnant women also have reasons to withhold information about their use of substances in pregnancy. Some states have mandatory reporting requirements with the possibility of incarceration in a minority of states. This may not only create a disincentive for disclosure, but possibly for treatment-seeking itself [22]. Women may also be concerned about prejudicial treatment and stigma from their physicians who should be their advocates, while pregnant youth may fear disclosure to family members and the possible consequences of such disclosure.

Third, SBIRT research and practice has traditionally focused on the more commonly used substances such as alcohol and tobacco, with relatively less focus

| Component | Goal | Approach |
|-----------|------|----------|
| Screening | To assess substance use and its severity | Patient-/computer-administered instrument or direct provider questions (see Figure 2.2) |
| Brief intervention | To increase intrinsic motivation to affect behavioral change (i.e. reduce or abstain from use) | 1–5 patient-centered counseling sessions lasting less than 15 minutes using principles of motivational interviewing (see Figure 2.5) |
| Referral to treatment | To provide those identified as needing more treatment access to specialty care | Warm handoff to specialized treatment (e.g. provider to provider phone call), which requires practitioner familiarity with community resources and systems of care |

**Figure 2.1** Components of screening, brief intervention, referral to treatment (SBIRT)

on illicit drugs [23]. This gap has become particularly apparent and troubling as rates of prescription drug misuse in pregnancy have risen steadily in recent years, leading to almost fivefold increases in the incidence of Neonatal Abstinence Syndrome (NAS) between 2000 and 2012 [24]. Recent literature has shown utility for SBIRT for illicit drug use during pregnancy [25].

## Screening

Screening for substance use should be universal, as SUDs occur in every socioeconomic class, racial and ethnic group. Moreover, screening based on "risk factors" such as late entry to PNC or prior poor birth outcome potentially leads to missed cases and can exacerbate stigma and stereotype [11]. Universal screening is recommended by many professional organizations, including ACOG [5], the AAP [26], the American Medical Association (AMA) [27], and the CDC [6]. Screening should be done at the first prenatal visit, and repeated at least every trimester for individuals who screen positive for past use. In addition, screening for tobacco use, at risk drinking, illicit drug use, and prescription drug misuse should occur on an annual basis as a part of routine well-woman care. Women should be asked at medical exams if they are planning to get pregnant in the next year, so that adequate contraception and preconception care can be provided.

Screening Summary:

- Screening for substance use should be done on all pregnant women at the first prenatal visit and subsequently throughout pregnancy on those women at higher risk;
- Screening can be done either by using a validated instrument with follow-up by the provider or by asking standardized questions during the interview;

- Screening should be nonjudgmental and questions should be open-ended;
- Urine toxicology testing should not be used in place of substance use screening questions.

Most of the studies looking at screening have focused on using instruments, such as TWEAK, TACE, 4P's, or Audit C. These instruments have the advantage of being validated and most are fairly sensitive. Also, preliminary screening can be done by anyone in the practice, with follow-up by the provider (Figure 2.2).

Barriers to implementing instrument-based screening include patient discomfort and lack of literacy, staff resistance due to time pressures, and organizational issues such as lack of administrative support [28]. Integration into practice flow can be eased by incorporation into electronic medical record systems (EMR) or by using a computer-based approach, which may diffuse the discomfort women feel in disclosing a behavior about which they are embarrassed, but this has not been compared to clinician administered screening in pregnant women [29]. All positive screens require follow-up by the provider.

To counteract some of the institutional barriers to instrument-based screening, some experts encourage simply asking three open-ended questions regarding use of tobacco, alcohol, and other drugs (The NIDA Quick Screen) [30]: In the past year how many times have you drunk more than four alcoholic drinks per day? Used tobacco? Taken illegal drugs or prescription drugs for nonmedical reasons? This screen needs to be validated in pregnancy. Women are also more likely to report lifetime use or use before pregnancy than they are to disclose use during pregnancy because of the risks and stigma involved. More important than the use of any specific screen is to be consistent and to ask the questions of everyone.

| Instrument | Substance | Validated in pregnancy | Subjects identified |
|---|---|---|---|
| CAGE [1]<br>– "Cut Down"<br>– "Annoyed"<br>– "Guilt"<br>– "Eye Opener" | Alcohol | No | At risk drinking |
| T-ACE [2]<br>– "Takes"<br>– "Annoyed"<br>– "Cut Down"<br>– "Eye Opener" | Alcohol | Yes | At risk drinking |
| TWEAK [3]<br>– "Tolerance"<br>– "Worry"<br>– "Eye Opener"<br>– "Amnesia"<br>– "Kut Down" | Alcohol | Yes | At risk drinking |
| 4Ps [4]<br>– Past<br>– Present<br>– Parents<br>– Partner | Any substance | Yes | Any affirmative is considered a positive screen |
| Substance Use Profile-Pregnancy [5] | Alcohol<br>Illicit drugs | Yes | Any drinking or illicit drugs |
| AUDIT-C | Alcohol | Yes | Any drinking |

*Modifications of the 4Ps screener are available, e.g. the 5Ps (adding smoking) and the 4P's Plus© [3] which is copyrighted and requires a yearly fee to use.

[1] Ewing J. A. Detecting alcoholism. The CAGE questionnaire. JAMA. 1984;252(14):1905–7.

[2] Sokol R. J., Martier S. S., Ager J. W. The T-ACE questions: practical prenatal detection of risk-drinking. *American Journal of Obstetrics and Gynecology*. 1989;160(4):863–8; discussion 8–70.

[3] Russell M. New assessment tools for risk drinking during pregnancy: T-ACE, TWEAK and others. *Alcohol Health & Research World*. 1994;18:55–61.

[4] Ewing H. *A Practical Guide to Intervention in Health and Social Services, with Pregnant and Postpartum Addicts and Alcoholics*. Martinez, CA: The Born Free Project, Contra Costa County Department of Health Services, 1990.

[5] Yonkers K. A., Gotman N., Kershaw T., Forray A., Howell H. B., Rounsaville B. J. Screening for prenatal substance use: development of the Substance Use Risk Profile-Pregnancy scale. *Obstetrics and Gynecology*. 2010;116(4):827–33.

**Figure 2.2** Examples of screening instruments

Regardless of which method is used and how the screening is delivered, it is essential that conversations around substance use be nonjudgmental. Prefacing screening with statements such as "I ask all my patients about substance use" can help normalize the enquiry and increase patient comfort with disclosure. The process of screening is only the first step in a conversation with the patient that may lead to treatment referral or provision of other treatment resources.

Urine drug testing is a common practice for many obstetricians and family practice physicians. It does have the advantage of detecting use in cases where the woman does not disclose her use and may help in diagnosing NAS. Toxicology testing is a useful adjunct for individuals in SUD treatment [31] and has utility at the time of delivery [6] in case of complications of pregnancy, where knowing the substance used informs management decisions. Toxicology testing of pregnant women also has a number of limitations and negative consequences and should therefore never be done without the woman's knowledge or consent. For example, it greatly increases the risk of legal or child welfare involvement, particularly in states with mandated reporting requirements that include mention of drug use during pregnancy. This places physicians in a difficult ethical position, and raises the likelihood that women will fail to disclose potential health risks or avoid recommended medical care [22]. Further,

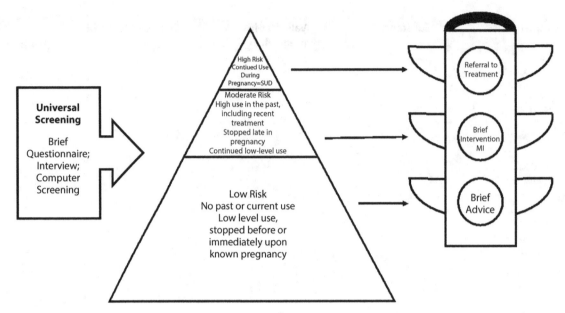

**Figure 2.3** Risk pyramid for substance use in pregnancy
SUD = substance use disorders

the reporting of drug use during pregnancy to child welfare – made more likely or even mandated as a result of positive toxicology – is strongly biased against racial and ethnic minorities [11], even following concerted efforts to prevent such bias [32]. A positive toxicology test also shows evidence of use, but does not provide any information about the nature or extent of that use; similarly, a negative test does not rule out substance use, which is often sporadic [15]. Additionally, the consequences of false positive results can be devastating to the woman and her family.

Finally, the use of toxicological testing for illicit drugs encourages a focus on substances such as cocaine, opiates, and marijuana that is not justified by their prevalence or the risk that they pose. Other substances such as tobacco and alcohol pose as much or more risk [33] and are far more prevalent [1]; similarly, other risk factors such as inadequate PNC, depression, or violence exposure present significant unique risks that should be acknowledged – and that is not amenable to toxicology testing. If drug testing is used, a discussion of all substances and medications taken is mandatory as it will allow the clinician to order the correct test(s). Many substances including synthetic opioids, such as oxycodone, fentanyl, buprenorphine, and some benzodiazepines [34], are not routinely captured by standard urine tests, and, if suspected, must

be ordered separately. In addition, regular urine drug screens do not pick up alcohol use, and tests for alcohol metabolites, such as ethyl glucuronide (ET-G) and ethyl sulfate (ET-S) are not routine, nor well studied in pregnant women. For these reasons, most specialty societies including ACOG, APA, and ASAM do not endorse using urine drug testing as a primary means to screen women for drug use during pregnancy.

Clinicians who do use urine drug testing should ensure that all positive drug tests are followed-up by confirmatory testing by mass spectrometry (MS). The health care provider should be aware of the potential for false-positive and false-negative results of urine toxicology for drug use, the typical urine drug metabolite detection times, and the legal and social consequences of a positive test result. It is incumbent on the health care provider, as part of the procedure in obtaining consent before testing, to provide information about the nature and purpose of the test to the patient and how the results will guide management [35]. Further discussion of urine drug screening will occur in Chapter 3.

The overarching purpose of screening for substance use is to stratify women into zones of risk given their pattern of use. The Expert Group on Perinatal Illicit Drug Abuse [36] developed the risk pyramid shown in Figure 2.3. The majority of women will fall into the low-risk zone (i.e. no past use of tobacco, alcohol, or

SBIRT flow

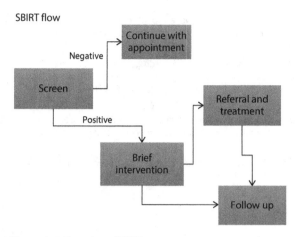

**Figure 2.4** Flow chart of SBIRT in practice

other drugs, or low levels of substance use that stopped prior to or immediately following knowledge of pregnancy) and will need only brief advice/reinforcement. Moderate-risk women are those who have used high quantities of (any) substances in the past (including those who have been recently treated for SUDs), those who stopped during pregnancy, and those with sporadic, low-level use during pregnancy. Per the consensus of the group, these are the women who benefit most from brief intervention (BI). Only about 4–5 percent of women will fall into the high-risk zone of continued use of illicit drugs during pregnancy [1]. Women in the high-risk zone meet criteria for SUD. While these women can benefit from BI, most need referral to specialized addiction treatment. Figure 2.4 illustrates the flow of SBIRT in clinical practice.

## Brief Intervention

Women who did not use substances prior to pregnancy or those who used at low-levels in the past and report cessation of all substance use (often due to pregnancy) are considered to be in the low-risk group. For this group, brief advice can be given. The simplest form of such intervention is reinforcement to remain abstinent (e.g. "That's great you do not use drugs or alcohol, as drug use has been shown to cause many complications in pregnancy and problems with your baby, and there is no safe amount of alcohol use in pregnancy" [37]). Providing written handouts to all women can reach women who are afraid to disclose use, but may be at risk and need treatment.

Individuals who screen positive for any substance use in pregnancy and fall into the moderate-risk group should receive a BI. This type of intervention is a patient-centered form of counseling using the principles of motivational interviewing (MI) to effect behavioral change. Motivational interviewing was first described by Miller in 1991 [38] and has been adapted to various interventions in health care settings [39]. The purpose of MI is not to "cure the patient," but to instill in her a desire to change by pointing out discrepancies between her current behavior and her future goals. This is facilitated in pregnancy because the overwhelming majority of women desire a healthy pregnancy and healthy baby. Principles of MI include using an empathetic counseling style, asking open-ended questions, developing rapport and trust, expressing empathy, and rolling with resistance. MI must be nonjudgmental and works best if the patient adopts the motivation and develops a plan to change her behavior [38].

For the provider, the three tasks of an effective BI are to: (1) provide feedback of personal responsibility (e.g. "As your doctor, I recommend you stop using cocaine for your health and the health of your baby, but it's your decision on what you want to do."); (2) listen and understand a patient's motivation for using one or more substances (e.g. "I hear that you use drugs to deal with the stress of your life at home"); and (3) explore other options to address patient's motivation for substance use (e.g. "Are there other ways you deal with stress in a more healthy way?"). Yet, the provider's objective is not to warn the patient as strong warning statements are often met with resistance from the patient. For example, stating: "Your baby could have a birth defect if you continue to drink alcohol" can be countered with: "I drank in my last pregnancy and that baby is fine." Resistance is a sign that the provider has pushed too hard. "Rolling with resistance" is a technique to redirect the conversation to a less threatening area. For example: "I'm not saying that your baby will definitely have a birth defect, but as your doctor, I'm concerned that your baby may be affected by your drinking. Babies who are exposed to alcohol in the womb can have lifelong medical and psychological problems."

Being judgmental, finger waiving, shaming, and/or using sarcasm are not effective ways of motivating people to implement behavioral changes. Finding a "hook" or reason for which the patient would like to change their harmful behavior is more effective (e.g. "How would your life be better if you didn't use

| Raise subject | • "Thank you for answering my questions – is it ok with you if we talk about your answers?"<br>• "Can you tell me more about your past/current drinking or drug use? What does a typical week look like?" |
|---|---|
| Provide feedback | • "Sometimes patients who give similar answers are continuing to use drugs or alcohol during their pregnancy."<br>• "I recommend all my pregnant patients not to use any alcohol or drugs, because of risk to you and to your baby." |
| Enhance motivation | • "What do you like and what are you concerned about when it comes to your substance use?"<br>• "On a scale of 0–10, how ready are you to avoid drinking/using altogether? Why that number and not a ____ (lower number)?" |
| Negotiate plan | • Summarize conversation. Then: "What steps do you think you can take to reach your goal of having a healthy pregnancy and baby?"<br>• "Can we schedule a date to check in about this next time?" |

**Figure 2.5** Components of a Brief Interview
Modified from SBIRTOregon.org [4]

opioids?"). One technique used often to discover this "hook" is to ask open-ended questions (e.g. "What do you like about ...?" or "What don't you like about ...?") followed by summary statements (e.g. "I hear that you smoke cigarettes to calm you down, but you don't like how much they cost and how they make you smell [i.e. reflecting the patient's own words], and you're worried about the effects they could have your baby. It sounds like having a healthy baby is very important to you.") Examples of language that can be used in a brief intervention are illustrated in Figure 2.5.

The BI can be followed with an oral or written "contract" in which the patient states what she plans on doing in order to reach readiness, abstinence, or interim goals toward eliminating substance use and the provider arranges for follow-up visits. This way, the patient remains responsible for her treatment and outcome, not the provider. Given that BIs are for patients with moderate-risk substance use, closer follow-up (generally every 2 weeks) is recommended. Patients who are unable to make any behavioral change or whose use increases during pregnancy should be referred for specialized addiction treatment. To help physicians implement SBIRT systems, the Oregon Health and Science University, with funding from the Substance Abuse and Mental Health Services Administration, developed an online portal (sbirtoregon.org) [40], which provides many excellent online resources including pocket cards and sample language that can be downloaded.

## Referral to Treatment

Only a minority of patients will screen into the high-risk category and require specialty treatment for substance use. These women are likely to meet criteria for having an SUD. Management of these women is the focus of the rest of this book. It is not the responsibility of the obstetric provider to deliver specialty treatment; however, his/her knowledge of appropriate referral resources is essential. Provision of addiction treatment in the same location as the PNC may be preferable as there is increased compliance with the behavioral health component and evidence of improved birth outcomes such as decreased rates of preterm labor and low birth weight following implementation of these services [41]. If such clinics are not available, good contacts for local specialty treatment services include state and local health departments, insurance preferred provider listings as well as national websites such as the SAMHSA treatment locator (www.findtreatment.samhsa.gov). The referral should be made via a "warm handoff," that is via direct communication between the PNC clinic and the SUD treatment site. Communication is key for the continued care of the pregnant patient in specialty substance use treatment. All patients should sign CFR 42 part B compliant release forms such that clinical information can be shared. The PNC provider can utilize BIs to support the SUD treatment progress during PNC, as there are some studies that show increased effect with increased dosages (better treatment outcomes with more MI sessions) [42].

## Barriers to SBIRT Implementation in Obstetric Practice

Reimbursement for the components of SBIRT exists through private insurers (CPT-codes 99408 and 99409) and Medicaid (H0049 and H0050). Payment for these codes do have relative value units (RVU) assigned to them, but not all payers will pay and there may be limitations on the number of SBIRT-related visits that qualify and are approved for reimbursement. In addition, they may not be reimbursed outside of the global OB reimbursement schedule. For reimbursement, screening/assessment instruments such as AUDIT and DAST should be used (SAMHSA www.samhsa.gov/sbirt/coding-reimbursement). Of note, SBIRT can be done by ancillary staff under the direction of the physician and added on to other E:M procedure codes. If the specific SBIRT code is not covered by insurance, generally a billable provider can use a corresponding E:M code for time-based counseling if the provider is the one providing the counseling. Generally, one would use the ICD-10 code for alcohol or specific SUD in order to obtain reimbursement.

Requirements of reporting pregnant women with SUD vary by state. The federal Child Abuse Prevention and Treatment Act (CAPTA) requires states to have policies and procedures in place to notify child protective services agencies of substance-exposed newborns and to establish a plan of safe care for newborns identified as being affected by illegal substance abuse or withdrawal symptoms resulting from prenatal drug exposure [43, 44]. Individual state statutes vary in what constitutes a substance-exposed newborn, when reporting should occur, and what constitutes a plan of safe care for the newborn. Specifics of each state statutes vary, but it is imperative that physicians caring for substance-using pregnant women know their individual state's requirements [43]. In practice, these policies, while seemingly important to ensure the safety of newborns/infants, often result in women being afraid to obtain PNC in fear that they may be reported to child welfare and lose custody of their infant as was seen in Chapter 1. Counseling patients that obtaining PNC and treatment for SUD improves their chances of maintaining custody can provide an important incentive for women to stay in treatment.

Many areas of the country, especially rural counties, lack treatment centers for SUD and especially services for women [45]. Transportation to urban areas for treatment, which often necessitates the woman being separated from her other children, represents a large barrier to treatment. Having more primary care providers certified in providing medication-assisted treatment with buprenorphine as well as expanding training in Addiction Medicine could help offset this treatment need, as could greater access to telemedicine and telepsychiatry [46].

Women who are accessing the health care system in any capacity (including treatment for SUD) should have their reproductive health care needs met at that time in order to help prevent substance-exposed pregnancies [47]. Substance use during pregnancy does not occur in isolation. It is often combined with a multitude of adverse life circumstances, such as poverty, interpersonal violence, psychiatric co-morbidity, and lack of access to adequate health care [48]. Women often enter medical care only when they are pregnant, and thus, it is important to address contraception during PNC, so that additional pregnancies are not substance-exposed. Barriers to both obtaining and using contraception that can effectively prevent pregnancy should be addressed. The postpartum period is a vulnerable time for relapse back to substance use [49, 50]. Continuing access to treatment and support services beyond the traditional 6-week postpartum period can help prevent relapse [51, 52]. Identifying risk factors for relapse and employing prevention techniques, such as dietary counseling, psychosocial care, and medical-assisted treatment can improve future pregnancy outcomes [48]. These services are ideally provided in a medical home environment, as the woman and infant remain at risk for the remainder of their lives, from her relapse to her SUD, which endangers not only her health, but also the health and safety of her entire family. Communication between the obstetric provider and the pediatric provider is imperative so that the infant can be provided with early interventions to identify and treat medical and behavioral problems, which can be lifelong and costly if not treated early.

## Summary

SBIRT is an important health intervention that should be integrated into PNC so to reduce the burden of both undiagnosed and untreated substance use in pregnancy. Identifying women with substance use and SUD during pregnancy allows providers to identify women at risk for having a substance-exposed newborn and tailor counseling and intervention to the women at risk. Pregnancy is the ultimate "teachable moment," when motivation for behavioral change is high.

Pregnancy is a state of individual biological and social transformation. From a public health perspective, it is a window of opportunity for addressing substance use, including SUDs as all pregnant women manifest interest in and care for the health of their baby-to-be. Therefore, most women can be helped to quit or cut back on substance use.

Given how common substance use is as well as the evidence supporting BIs in reducing such use during the perinatal period, the expert group concluded that universal screening, ideally at PNC intake, is key to addressing substance use in pregnancy; of note, universal screening is recommended by ACOG [5], the American Academy of Pediatrics [26], and the AMA [27]. Screening will determine an individual's risk stratification – low-risk women should receive brief advice, those with moderate-risk should receive a BI, whereas those who are high-risk need referral to specialty care. Patients who are unable to make any behavioral change or whose use increases during pregnancy should be referred for specialized addiction treatment. Irrespective of risk stratification and where they are during the SBIRT process, it is imperative that pregnant and postpartum women who use one or more substances be treated with respect and compassion by their providers.

# References

1. Substance Abuse and Mental Health Services Administration, Results from the 2013 National Survey on Drug Use and Health: Summary of National Findings, NSDUH Series H-48, HHS Publication No. (SMA) 14-4863. Rockville, MD: Substance Abuse and Mental Health Services Administration, 2014.

2. Viteri O. A., Soto E. E., Bahado-Singh R. O., et al. Fetal anomalies and long-term effects associated with substance abuse in pregnancy: a literature review. *American Journal of Perinatology.* 2015;32(5):405–16.

3. Substance Abuse and Mental Health Services Administration (2014) *Prevention of Substance Abuse and Mental Illness.* www.samhsa.gov/prevention. Accessed 13 April 2015.

4. Patrick S. W., Schumacher R. E., Benneyworth B. D., et al. Neonatal abstinence syndrome and associated health care expenditures: United States, 2000–2009. *Journal of the American Medical Association.* 2012;307(18):1934–40.

5. American College of Obstetricians and Gynecologists. At-risk drinking and illicit drug use: ethical issues in obstetric and gynecologic practice. ACOG Committee Opinion No. 422. *Obstetrics and Gynecology.* 2008;112:1449–60.

6. Jones H. E., Deppen K., Hudak M. L., et al. Clinical care for opioid-using pregnant and postpartum women: the role of obstetric providers. *American Journal of Obstetrics and Gynecology.* 2014;210(4):302–10.

7. Madras B. K. C. W., Avula D., Stegbauer T., Stein J. B., Clark H. W. Screening, brief interventions, referral to treatment (SBIRT) for illicit drug and alcohol use at multiple healthcare sites: comparison at intake and six months. *Drug and Alcohol Dependence.* 2009; 99(1–3):280–95.

8. U.S. Preventative Services Task Force. Counseling and interventions to prevent tobacco use and tobacco-caused disease in adults and pregnant women: U.S. Preventive Services Task Force reaffirmation recommendation statement. *Annals of Internal Medicine* 2009;150(8):551–5.

9. Jonas D. E., Garbutt J. C., Amick H. R., et al. Behavioral counseling after screening for alcohol misuse in primary care: a systematic review and meta-analysis for the U.S. Preventive Services Task Force. *Annals of Internal Medicine.* 2012;157(9): 645–54.

10. ACOG Committee on Ethics. ACOG Committee Opinion No. 422: at-risk drinking and illicit drug use: ethical issues in obstetric and gynecologic practice. *Obstetrics & Gynecology.* 2008;112(6):1449–60.

11. Chasnoff I. J., Landress H. J., Barrett M. E. The prevalence of illicit-drug or alcohol use during pregnancy and discrepancies in mandatory reporting in Pinellas County, Florida. *The New England Journal of Medicine.* 1990;322(17):1202–6.

12. Mengel M. B., Searight H. R., Cook K. Preventing alcohol-exposed pregnancies. *Journal of the American Board of Family Medicine: JABFM.* 2006;19(5):494–505.

13. Anderson B. L., Dang E. P., Floyd R. L., et al. Knowledge, opinions, and practice patterns of obstetrician-gynecologists regarding their patients' use of alcohol. *Journal of Addiction Medicine.* 2010;4(2):114–21.

14. Ewing J. A. Detecting alcoholism. The CAGE questionnaire. *Journal of the American Medical Association.* 1984;252(14):1905–7.

15. American College of Obstetricians and Gynecologists. Substance abuse reporting and pregnancy: the role of the obstetrician-gynecologist committee opinion 473. *Obstetrics and Gynecology.* 2011;117(1):200–1.

16. O'Brien P. L. Performance measurement: a proposal to increase use of SBIRT and decrease alcohol consumption during pregnancy. *Maternal and Child Health Journal.* 2014;18(1):1–9.

17. Garg M., Garrison L., Leeman L., et al. Validity of self-reported drug use information among pregnant women. *Maternal and Child Health Journal.* 2016;20:41–7.

18. Grekin E. R., Svikis D. S., Lam P., et al. Drug use during pregnancy: validating the Drug Abuse Screening Test against physiological measures. *Psychology of Addictive Behaviors.* 2010;24(4): 719–23.

19. Markovic N., Ness R. B., Cefilli D., et al. Substance use measures among women in early pregnancy. *American Journal of Obstetrics and Gynecology.* 2000;183(3):627–32.

20. Ostrea E. M., Jr., Knapp D. K., Tannenbaum L., et al. Estimates of illicit drug use during pregnancy by maternal interview, hair analysis, and meconium analysis. *Journal of Pediatrics* 2001;138(3):344–8.

21. Ostrea E. M., Jr., Brady M., Gause S., Raymundo A. L., Stevens M. Drug screening of newborns by meconium analysis: a large-scale, prospective, epidemiologic study. *Pediatrics.* 1992;89(1):107–13.

22. Poland M. L., Dombrowski M. P., Ager J. W., Sokol R. J. Punishing pregnant drug users: enhancing the flight from care. *Drug and Alcohol Dependence.* 1993;31(3):199–203.

23. Farr S. L., Hutchings Y. L., Ondersma S. J., Creanga A. A. Brief interventions for illicit drug use among peripartum women. *American Journal of Obstetrics and Gynecology.* 2014;211:336–43.

24. Patrick S. W., Davis M. M., Lehmann C. U., Cooper W. O. Increasing incidence and geographic distribution of neonatal abstinence syndrome: United States 2009 to 2012. *Journal of Perinatology: Official Journal of the California Perinatal Association.* 2015;35(8):650–5.

25. Farr S. L., Hutchings Y. L., Ondersma S. J., Creanga A. A. Brief interventions for illicit drug use among peripartum women. *American Journal of Obstetrics and Gynecology.* 2014;211(4):336–43.

26. Levy S. J., Kokotailo P. K. Substance use screening, brief intervention, and referral to treatment for pediatricians. *Pediatrics.* 2011;128(5):e1330–40.

27. Blum L. N., Nielsen N. H., Riggs J. A. Alcoholism and alcohol abuse among women: report of the Council on Scientific Affairs. American Medical Association. *Journal of Women's Health/the Official Publication of the Society for the Advancement of Women's Health Research.* 1998;7(7):861–71.

28. Bentley S. M., Melville J. L., Berry B. D., Katon W. J. Implementing a clinical and research registry in obstetrics: overcoming the barriers. *General Hospital Psychiatry.* 2007;29(3):192–8.

29. Tzilos G. K., Sokol R. J., Ondersma S. J. A randomized phase I trial of a brief computer-delivered intervention for alcohol use during pregnancy. *Journal of Women's Health (2002).* 2011;20(10):1517–24.

30. National Institute on Drug Abuse, The NIDA Quick Screen. *Resource Guide: Screening for Drug Use in General Medical Settings.* National Institute on Drug Abuse, March 2012. Available from: www.drugabuse.gov/publications/resource-guide-screening-drug-use-in-general-medical-settings/nida-quick-screen.

31. Jacobs W., DuPont R., Gold M. S. Drug testing and the DSM-IV. *Psychiatric Annals.* 2000;30:583–8.

32. Roberts S., Zahnd E., Sufrin C., Armstrong M. A. Does adopting a prenatal substance use protocol reduce racial disparities in CPS reporting related to maternal drug use? A California case study. *Journal of Perinatology.* 2015;35(2):146–50.

33. Janisse J., Bailey B., Ager J., Sokol R. Alcohol, tobacco, cocaine, and marijuana use: relative contributions to preterm delivery and fetal growth restriction. *Substance Abuse* 2014;35(1):60–7.

34. Tenore P. Advanced urine toxicology testing. *Journal of Addictive Diseases.* 2010;29:436–48.

35. American College of Obstetricians and Gynecologists. Patient testing: ethical issues in selection and counseling. ACOG Committee Opinion No. 363. *Obstetrics & Gynecology.* 2007;109:1021–3.

36. Wright T. E., Terplan M., Ondersma S. J., et al. The role of screening, brief intervention, and referral to treatment in the perinatal period. *American Journal of Obstetrics and Gynecology.* 2016;215(5):539–47.

37. Yonkers K. A., Forray A., Howell H. B., et al. Motivational enhancement therapy coupled with cognitive behavioral therapy versus brief advice: a randomized trial for treatment of hazardous substance use in pregnancy and after delivery. *General Hospital Psychiatry.* 2012;34(5):439–49.

38. Miller W. R., Rollnick S. *Motivational Interviewing: Preparing People to Change Addictive Behavior.* 3rd ed. New York: The Guildford Press; 1991 September 7, 2012.

39. Rollnick S., Miller W. R., Butler C. C. *Motivational Interviewing in Health Care: Helping Patients Change Behavior.* 1st ed. New York: The Guilford Press; 2007 November 7, 2007.

40. Oregon Health and Science University. Department of Family Medicine. *SBIRT Oregon.* 2016. Available from: www.sbirtoregon.org/.

41. Armstrong M. A., Gonzales Osejo V., Lieberman L., et al. Perinatal substance abuse intervention in obstetric clinics decreases adverse neonatal outcomes. *Journal of Perinatology: Official Journal of the California Perinatal Association.* 2003;23(1):3–9.

42. Burke B. L., Arkowitz H., Menchola M. The efficacy of motivational interviewing: a meta-analysis of controlled clinical trials. *Journal of Consulting and Clinical Psychology.* 2003;71(5):843–61.

43. Child Welfare Information Gateway. (2012). *Parental Drug Abuse as Child Abuse.* Washington, DC: U.S. Department of Health and Human Services, Children's Bureau.

44. National Center on Substance Abuse and Child Welfare: Substance Abuse and Mental Health Services Administration. Available from: www.ncsacw.samhsa.gov/aboutus/default.aspx.

45. Terplan M., Longinaker N., Appel L. Women-centered drug treatment services and need in the United States, 2002–2009. *American Journal of Public Health.* 2015;105(11):e50-4.

46. Sigmon S. C. Access to treatment for opioid dependence in rural America: challenges and future directions. *JAMA Psychiatry.* 2014;71(4): 359–60.

47. Terplan M., Hand D. J., Hutchinson M., Salisbury-Afshar E., Heil S. H. Contraceptive use and method choice among women with opioid and other substance use disorders: a systematic review. *Preventive Medicine.* 2015;80:23–31.

48. Wright T. E., Schuetter R., Fombonne E., Stephenson J., Haning W. F., 3rd. Implementation and evaluation of a harm-reduction model for clinical care of substance using pregnant women. *Harm Reduction Journal.* 2012;9(1):5.

49. Forray A., Merry B., Lin H., Ruger J. P., Yonkers K. A. Perinatal substance use: a prospective evaluation of abstinence and relapse. *Drug and Alcohol Dependence.* 2015;150:147–55.

50. El-Mohandes A. A., El-Khorazaty M. N., Kiely M., Gantz M. G. Smoking cessation and relapse among pregnant African-American smokers in Washington, DC. *Maternal and Child Health Journal.* 2011;15 Suppl 1:S96–105.

51. Niccols A., Milligan K., Sword W., et al. Integrated programs for mothers with substance abuse issues: a systematic review of studies reporting on parenting outcomes. *Harm Reduction Journal.* 2012;9:14.

52. Barlow A., Mullany B., Neault N., et al. Paraprofessional-delivered home-visiting intervention for American Indian teen mothers and children: 3-year outcomes from a randomized controlled trial. *The American Journal of Psychiatry.* 2015;172(2):154–62.

# Substance Use Assessment during Pregnancy

Jacquelyn Starer and Carl Christensen

Universal screening for substance use disorders (SUDs) will identify many, but not all, pregnant women with SUDs. Stigma, shame, and fear of real and perceived harms from disclosure will cause many women to hide or deny their substance use during pregnancy. Other women have a more advanced disease and have spent years learning how to hide their addictions in order to protect their use.

Therefore, assessment of SUDs during pregnancy will include the management of both those women identified during the screening process and those not yet identified. Those women identified during the screening process will need appropriate care and ongoing assessment of abstinence versus continued or intermittent drug use.

The women not yet identified may have risk factors or clinical signs and symptoms of substance use and the practitioner will need to be able to recognize and address these concerns as they arise. Additionally, universal screening tools should be repeated as the pregnancy progresses, at least once per trimester and again on labor and delivery. The casual or intermittent user of drugs or alcohol will often be the most difficult to identify because there will be fewer signs and symptoms. These patients may be able to time their use around the times of their pre-natal visits. Ongoing education for patients as part of routine counseling regarding the consequences of drugs and alcohol will be helpful in reducing use among the casual user.

## Pregnant Women with SUDs Not Identified with Initial Screening

Women with appropriate opioid use such as those taking prescribed opioids via prescriptions will be more likely to be identified during the screening process than the woman who is misusing prescription medications or using illicit drugs. For those who do not report taking prescribed opioids, they should be identifiable using the state prescription monitoring programs

(PMPs) [1]. All physicians should register for their state PMP programs [2]. Patients who may not be identified via a state PMP could include women who are being prescribed and filling their prescriptions out of state. Some patients may be using online pharmacies but this should be considered misuse unless the patient received the prescription from a regular caregiver.

Out-of-state prescriptions can be a particular problem in border areas. Some states have agreements with bordering states to share information across state lines in their prescription monitoring databases. Physicians should familiarize themselves with their own states' PMP and whether information from neighboring states is included. A large number of states do share their PMP data and physicians should stay current on the availability of this information in their state and which states participate in PMP data sharing [3]. If a patient is using a prescribed opioid for pain as directed by a legitimate prescriber and does not disclose this information to her obstetrician, this could be considered a red flag for SUD, but also could be due to fear of reporting to child welfare. This should be addressed in a nonjudgmental manner, and confidentiality should be assured.

Women taking prescription opioid medications can be considered to have an opioid use disorder (OUD) if they take more than prescribed or use in an aberrant pattern. Additionally, any woman taking prescription opioid medication that was not prescribed for her should be considered to have an OUD or to be at high risk for an OUD. This includes women borrowing opioid medication from friends or family.

Unfortunately, there are some physicians and other prescribers who have overprescribed and who have contributed to the current epidemic of opioid use. The medical world is at a crossroads regarding the ongoing practice of long-term use of high dose opioid medication for chronic pain conditions [4]. If a woman has been chronically prescribed unusually high doses of an opioid, she will typically have a diagnosis to support that use, will become dependent on that dose, and both she and her physician may be very resistant to the suggestion that her use is inappropriate or that other modalities may be available. The fact that she has a physician supporting her use is extremely validating to that patient. It is inappropriate to suggest that this patient have her medication changed to methadone or buprenorphine without further assessment. Doing so labels her as having an OUD. Being treated as a patient with an OUD rather than a patient with chronic pain puts her in a different treatment milieu, which could be alternatively helpful or harmful. This will be a very difficult and frustrating situation for the obstetrical care team. Instead of labeling the patient with an OUD, using harm reduction principles and "meeting the patient where she's at," can continue the patient's engagement in prenatal care and other treatment, which is imperative for the best pregnancy outcomes. It is important to individualize treatment to best meet the needs of that patient, in coordination with her other prescribers and consultation with addiction medicine specialists.

## Risk Factors for SUD

Recognized signs and symptoms that represent a risk of SUD will generally fail to be all-inclusive and will also be nondiagnostic. When interviewing a patient at risk for SUD, there can be subtleties that suggest the patient may be avoiding disclosure. Patients with SUDs may minimize or rationalize their drug or alcohol use, they may exhibit behaviors that discourage further questioning such as anger or irritability, they might lie, and they might have personal denial of the consequences of their use.

Whether the 4Ps [5] are used as a screening tool or not, the last two questions of that tool are useful to keep in mind:

**4Ps for Substance Abuse:**
1. Have you ever used drugs or alcohol during **Pregnancy?**
2. Have you had a problem with drugs or alcohol in the **Past?**
3. Does your **Partner** have a problem with drugs or alcohol?
4. Do you consider one of your **Parents** to be an addict or alcoholic?

Family and partner history are not only risk factors, but are also a good way to initiate a conversation. Patients are often more comfortable discussing drug and alcohol use among others than in discussing their own use. This discussion can lead to better rapport if the information is discussed in an empathic and nonjudgmental style.

There are many psychosocial factors that may be considered risk factors for substance use. These include an unstable job or educational history as demonstrated by frequent job changes or interruptions in education. High-risk behaviors include multiple sexual partners, history of sexually transmitted diseases, multiple pregnancy terminations, and working in strip or nude clubs or erotic dance clubs. Relationship problems such as intimate partner violence, history of childhood physical or sexual abuse, current marital dysfunction, and other social behaviors such as isolation, loss of friendships, distance from family members, and lack of interest or participation in hobbies or recreational activities can all be risk factors or warning signs of drug or alcohol use. Patients with chronic pain syndromes may be at risk for substance use in order to self-medicate their symptoms [6].

Behaviors and activities leading to legal problems are red flags for drug and alcohol use. This includes prostitution, violent behavior, assaults, DWI history, child custody problems, theft, and the more obvious crimes such as drug possession or sale. Frequent accidents, injuries, and falls can be additional signposts.

A thorough psychiatric history should be taken and patients should be observed for symptoms of depression, anxiety, post-traumatic stress disorder, sleep disturbance, memory problems, difficulty concentrating, and suicidal ideation.

During pregnancy, women with SUDs may initiate prenatal care late or not at all, have frequent missed appointments, behave erratically, or show signs of sedation, euphoria, intoxication, or withdrawal. Poor weight gain and poor nutrition can accompany substance use. The obstetrical history may also suggest risk factors, such as placental abruption, premature birth, low gestational size, and neonatal withdrawal syndrome in the infant.

## Physical Signs of Drug and Alcohol Use

If drug use is parenteral, a thorough examination of the skin may reveal needle marks, track marks, signs of acute or chronic inflammation, evidence of "skin popping" or intradermal injection, cellulitis, and abscesses [7]. Parenteral use also increased the risk of co-existing

HIV, Hepatitis B and C, bacterial endocarditis, and osteomyelitis. Histamine release from opioids causes itching and scratching, which can cause excoriation.

Opioid use causes meiosis, and withdrawal causes mydriasis. Excessive opioid use causes sedation, nodding off, and respiratory depression but mild intoxication will induce euphoria, talkativeness (soap boxing) [8], increased sociability, and stimulation with associated increased activity. These periods of good mood and activity may be difficult for a clinician to recognize as an opioid effect. Opioid withdrawal symptoms also include anxiety, restlessness, irritability, yawning, rhinorrhea, lacrimation, nausea, vomiting, sweating, chills, and gooseflesh (piloerection).

Opioid users will often use other drugs (polysubstance use) and this will confound the clinical picture. Signs and symptoms of other drug or alcohol use include alcohol on the breath, ascites, an enlarged liver, nasal ulcers or a perforated septum, poor dental health, obesity or cachexia, abnormal gait, tremor, slurred speech, change in pupil size, blackouts, accidental overdoses, other liver or gastrointestinal problems, conjunctival injection (bloodshot eyes), hyperphagia or anorexia, elevated blood pressure, tachycardia, chest pain, transient ischemic attacks, restlessness, sweating, and tremor – from withdrawal or stimulant intoxication [6].

# Clinical Assessment of SUDs during Pregnancy

All pregnant women with an identified SUD should have a comprehensive medical history and physical examination including laboratory testing and a through psychosocial assessment. All elements of routine prenatal care should be provided. Consultation, communication, and coordination with an addiction specialist is recommended as the care of these patients can require multiple additional visits, phone calls, follow-up, and laboratory testing that may be beyond the capability and expertise of many obstetrical practices.

Mental health disorders, which often co-exist with SUDs, should be referred for appropriate psychiatric evaluation and treatment. It is best to find specialized psychiatric providers experienced in the care of pregnant women in order to maximize the use of nonpharmacologic treatments and to avoid or minimize the use of psychoactive medications such as benzodiazepines. Significant psychiatric conditions will require medication treatment. These conditions will be addressed in Chapter 4.

Monitoring abstinence from drugs and alcohol is best done through a combination of open patient communication as well as observation of signs and symptoms and behavioral patterns. Toxicology testing can be a useful adjunct in treatment settings, but should only be done with the written consent of the pregnant patient for the reasons discussed in Chapter 2. Drug testing will be discussed in detail later in this chapter.

# Monitoring Pregnant Patients on Opioid Agonist Treatment (OAT)

Treatment of pregnant women with OUDs with opioid agonist medication throughout the pregnancy is the gold standard of care. A small percentage of women who have been either prescribed opioid pain medication or who have a mild OUD and are highly motivated may be candidates for medically supervised withdrawal (MSW) under the care of an addiction medicine specialist. MSW undertaken by the obstetrician should be done as part of a comprehensive substance use program and caution should be taken that all laws regarding opioid treatment are followed. Long-term intensive behavioral treatment is needed for successful outcomes with MSW during pregnancy, otherwise rates of relapse to harmful substance use with often deadly consequences is all too common [9].

The two opioid agonists currently approved for treatment of OUDs in the United States are buprenorphine and methadone. Treatment with these medications is usually referred to as Medication Assisted Treatment (MAT) or Opioid Agonist Treatment (OAT). Details of MAT/OAT will be addressed in Chapter 10.

Assessment of pregnant women receiving MAT requires communication with the MAT prescribers, with signed CFR 42 part B compliant release forms. Participation by a woman in an MAT program does not necessarily mean she is abstinent from illicit opioid use or other drug or alcohol use. Therefore, it is necessary to periodically review the woman's success or address her struggles in treatment with the addiction treatment team.

Physicians and clinicians working in MAT programs are identified as addiction treatment providers and, as such, can only communicate with others, including other health care providers and obstetrical care providers, after the patient has signed a specialized consent form that complies with the law, specifically CFR 42 part B. Addiction providers will have CFR 42 part B compliant release forms. All pregnant patients known to be receiving these medications should be asked to sign a CFR 42 part B compliant release form allowing communication between the obstetrical team and the MAT team.

Not all pregnant women who are receiving MAT will be willing to sign a release form. This may be due to fear of child custody issues or other concerns. It is possible that a pregnant woman may never reveal her MAT with her obstetrical team. This is particularly true for women receiving methadone, which is always dispensed from a specialized federally licensed Opioid Treatment Program (OTP) in the United States. Although the methadone is prescribed, it is not dispensed by a pharmacy and, therefore, the methadone will not appear on a state PMP, or Prescription Monitoring Program, review. With appropriate and persistent counseling done by the OTP about the importance of disclosure of the treatment in order to provide the best care of her and her infant, hopefully most women will provide consent.

Pregnant women being prescribed buprenorphine for an OUD may be treated in an OTP, in a practice or clinic specializing in buprenorphine treatment, or in a private medical practice office. A CFR 42 part B compliant release form is also required in order to communicate with buprenorphine prescribers.

Obstetricians should contact the MAT prescribers if there are concerns of excessive medication effect or other signs and symptoms of drug use. Patients who are using additional drugs or medication may do so after they have seen their MAT prescriber and the MAT prescriber may not be aware of these signs or symptoms. There are many sedating medications now being misused by patients in order to augment the effects of their treatment medications. These drugs may not show up on a drug test because they are not all uniformly recognized as drugs of abuse. Common medications used in this fashion are clonidine [10], gabapentin, promethazine [11], and muscle relaxants, in addition to the commonly abused medications such as benzodiazepines, sleeping medications, and barbiturates.

## Toxicology and Biomarkers as Assessment Tools

Laboratory testing may be used as screening tools as discussed in the previous chapter but become particularly important when assessing patients identified as having an SUD and monitoring those patients in treatment for an SUD.

Criteria developed for screening tests are also relevant in determining which tools and tests to utilize for assessment and monitoring. In order to qualify as a screening test, the following criteria should be met [12]:

The screening program should respond to a recognized need.

1. The objectives of screening should be defined at the outset.
2. There should be a defined target population.
3. There should be scientific evidence of screening program effectiveness.
4. The program should integrate education, testing, clinical services, and program management.
5. There should be quality assurance, with mechanisms to minimize potential risks of screening.
6. The program should ensure informed choice, confidentiality, and respect for autonomy.
7. The program should promote equity and access to screening for the entire target population.
8. Program evaluation should be planned from the outset.
9. The overall benefits of screening should outweigh the harm.

Written, informed consent from the patient is strongly advised when performing laboratory testing for screening, assessment, or monitoring of patients at risk for SUDs [13].

There are also ethical considerations involved in screening or testing, especially with regards to criteria 9 (benefits vs harm). In screening or testing pregnant women for SUD, the harm caused may involve legal complications and loss of custody.

The ethical principles involved in screening include autonomy/informed consent, nonmaleficence, and beneficence. Autonomy refers to the capacity to make a rational, informed decision. Beneficence and nonmaleficence are often considered together, whereby beneficence implies "doing the right thing" for the patient and non-maleficence is "do no harm." In drug testing the pregnant patient, this argument often comes down to: should the pregnant patient sign an informed consent prior to drug testing?

The crux of the "informed consent" argument relates to the case of Ferguson v. Charleston, involving a pregnant patient whose urine drug screens results were turned over to the police, rather than referred for counseling. This was eventually found to be a violation of the 4th Amendment and that beneficence did not apply [13]. Currently, at many institutions, urine drug screen results are not available to outside parties due to HIPAA, and CFR part 42, unless there is a subpoena or release of information obtained. The same warnings apply to the Prescription Drug Management Programs (PDMP).

# Laboratory Testing for SUD

Laboratory testing consists primarily of urine drug **screening** (UDS) which are immunoassays with significant rates of false positives or false negatives. UDS may or may not be followed by confirmatory testing or urine drug **testing** (UDT) (gas chromatography/mass spectroscopy or liquid chromatography), depending on the protocols involved. It is important to confirm with your lab or testing entity that confirmatory testing involves these more specific techniques and does not refer simply to a repeat of the original immunoassay. Urine drug screening may also be done as Point of Care Testing (POCT) in the office or ED setting and gives immediate results. POCT involves urine dipstick testing as opposed to a laboratory analysis. The following general concerns apply:

a. Urine drug screening, especially when done in the office setting, has a high false positive and negative rate, is not allowed by governmental (DOT) agencies, and does not identify the specific drug (i.e., identifies only drug classes such as benzodiazepines as opposed to the specific drug such as alprazolam vs clonazepam). Thus, there is no way to know whether the patient is taking the prescribed medication or another medication. Many drugs, i.e., buprenorphine, are missing from standard UDS cups. In some cases, only "natural" opioids (codeine, morphine, and heroin) are identified.

b. Urine drug testing involving confirmation are more accurate (fewer false positives and false negatives) but are much more expensive; the practitioner should make the patient aware of the potential for being billed.

c. With either testing method, needed drug testing may need to be specifically requested; i.e., fentanyl, methadone, buprenorphine/naloxone, Kratom, synthetic drugs such as K2.

d. In order to prevent false positive results, the drug concentration should be "normalized" to a creatinine of 100 (u100). This is done by taking the drug concentration, multiplying by 100, and dividing by the creatinine (drug ng/ml × 100)/creatinine. This allows the practitioner to monitor a declining drug level to determine if drug use has stopped. This has been validated primarily for THC but can be extrapolated to other drugs [14].

e. Urine screening for alcohol is notoriously difficult, because it is cleared so rapidly and the patient has to be "under the influence" at the time of the test, thus heavy use the day or night before could be missed. To better allow identification and monitoring of alcohol use, the urine can be tested for ethyl glucuronide (ETG) and ethyl sulfate (ETS), which are both hepatic metabolites of ethanol. There have been multiple reports of false positives for this test at low levels, including with use hand sanitizer, mouthwash, and foods. Specific conditions for testing for ETG and ETS include:

i. A cutoff of 250 ng/ml or greater should be used. According to SAMHSA, values greater than 1,000 ng/ml are not due to extraneous use.

ii. The value should be normalized to a creatinine of 100 (see above).

iii. In borderline cases, additional testing can be done (see below).

f. To prevent tampering (adding water), adulteration (adding a chemical to the urine), or substitution (nonurine), the following should be confirmed by the testing method. This is included routinely on most commercial POCT tests and by licensed drug testing laboratories:

i. Temperature (90–100 F)

ii. Creatinine: >20 mg/ml

iii. Specific gravity: greater than 1.003 (can be skipped if creatinine is normal)

iv. Adulterants: <200 ug/ml.
    Additionally, certain collection techniques will reduce the risk of urine tampering. These techniques include inspection of the patient and removal of all outer garments or bags, turning off the water supply in the collection room, coloring the toilet water, removal of all soaps and cleaning agents, and sometimes may involve observed donation if deemed necessary.

g. Opioid use can consist of either prescription pill misuse and/or heroin use. Heroin (di-acetylmorphine) is rapidly metabolized to

23

6-mono-acetylmorphine (6MAM) and then to morphine. The presence of 6MAM is confirmatory for heroin, while the unexplained presence of morphine, greater than 300 ng/ml, is concerning. Codeine is also seen with heroin and may be metabolized to morphine.

h. Interpretation of urine drug screens can be notoriously difficult, and patients should not be accused of using a nonprescribed medication unless one is familiar with the drug's metabolism. For example, a patient prescribed hydrocodone (Norco®) may test positive for hydromorphone (Dilaudid®). A patient who tests positive for codeine (Tylenol #3®) may test positive for morphine; and a patient prescribed Oxycodone may test positive for oxymorphone (Opana®). Most commercial laboratories have an MRO (Medical Review Officer) available for questions regarding drug identification.

i. Additional testing techniques: two additional techniques are available, although not widely used in pregnancy. These are the phosphatidyl ethanol (PEth) and hair analysis. The PEth test is used to detect alcohol use over a longer period of time. It is a blood based test and can be done any time needed and goes back over several weeks. Hair testing, which typically goes back over 90 days or more, requires a 2 or more week wait before testing and is not as comprehensive as urine testing. Hair testing has other drawbacks including lack of standardization. Drugs concentrate differently in processed hair and hair of different ethnicities (e.g. higher concentrations in darker hair).

## Making a Diagnosis

Once a patient has screened "positive" for an SUD, either as part of universal screening, laboratory screening, or other assessment methods, it is critical that a diagnosis of SUD not be made without an addiction evaluation. This will normally consist of a detailed interview, history and focused physical examination with additional laboratory tests.

The criteria used for making a diagnosis of an SUD are defined in the Diagnostic Service Manual criteria, now in its 5th edition. This edition has combined two previous diagnoses: abuse and dependence. The abuse criteria (typically risky use, failure to perform at work/school/interpersonal relationships, and recurrent legal problems) have been combined with the dependence

---

**Opioid Use Disorder Criteria:**

A minimum of 2–3 criteria is required for a mild substance use disorder diagnosis, while 4–5 is moderate, and 6–7 is severe (APA, 2013). Opioid Use Disorder is specified instead of Substance Use Disorder, if opioids are the drug of abuse.

1. Taking the opioid in larger amounts and for longer than intended
2. Wanting to cut down or quit but not being able to do it
3. Spending a lot of time obtaining the opioid
4. Craving or a strong desire to use opioids
5. Repeatedly unable to carry out major obligations at work, school, or home due to opioid use
6. Continued use despite persistent or recurring social or interpersonal problems caused or made worse by opioid use
7. Stopping or reducing important social, occupational, or recreational activities due to opioid use
8. Recurrent use of opioids in physically hazardous situations
9. Consistent use of opioids despite acknowledgment of persistent or recurrent physical or psychological difficulties from using opioids
10. *Tolerance as defined by either a need for markedly increased amounts to achieve intoxication or desired effect or markedly diminished effect with continued use of the same amount (does not apply for diminished effect when used appropriately under medical supervision).
11. *Withdrawal manifesting as either characteristic syndrome or the substance is used to avoid withdrawal (does not apply when used appropriately under medical supervision).

*This criterion is not considered to be met for those individuals taking opioids solely under appropriate medical supervision.

**Figure 3.1** DSM5 criteria for opioid use disorders

*Source*: APA. *Diagnostic and Statistical Manual of Mental Disorders*, 5th ed. Arlington: American Psychiatric Association, 2013.

---

(tolerance and withdrawal) criteria. The previous criterion for recurrent legal problems has been removed and "craving," an important feature of addiction, added. The criteria are then divided into Mild (similar to DSM IV Abuse), Moderate, and Severe (similar to DSM IV Dependence).

There are 4 categories for the DSM V:

- Impaired Control (4 criteria)
- Social Impairment (3 criteria)
- Risky Use (2 criteria)
- Pharmacological Criteria (2 criteria)

The entire DSM V criteria are listed in Figure 3.1. It should be kept in mind that a single episode, i.e., one positive urine drug screen, one DWI conviction, is not sufficient to make a DSM V diagnosis. A "recurrent" pattern is required.

To make a diagnosis of mild SUD, two criteria are required; for a moderate SUD, four to five; and for a severe SUD, six or more.

There are additional diagnostic descriptions, including "early remission" (more than 3 months), "sustained remission" (more than 12 months), and "partial" remission (not all criteria complied with). Note that "craving" is not considered when determining whether or not a patient is in remission.

## Level of Treatment

If a diagnosis of SUD is not made, then no treatment is recommended. However, the evaluator may also find a situation of "risky drinking" that exceeds safe drinking limits for women (in the case of pregnancy, none), in which case counseling and education is recommended. If risky drinking (any drinking) continues during pregnancy, then re-assessment is warranted. If a diagnosis of mild, moderate, or severe SUD, then a "level of care" of treatment should be recommended.

In the past, treatment was often recommended as "one size fits all"; typically, that meant the treatment program that the evaluator/therapist was most familiar with. Driven by financial considerations and lack of resources, a set of guidelines, published by the American Society of Addiction Medicine (now known as the ASAM criteria) [15], established what is known as "levels of care":

- Level 0: counseling for a lack of DSM diagnosis (i.e., risky drinking)
- Level 1: outpatient therapy (typically less than three times a week or less than 9 hours a week)
- Level 2: intensive outpatient therapy (three or more times a week, 9 or more hours a week, may also involve daily visits or Partial Hospitalization)
- Level 3: residential treatment (typically 30 days or longer)
- Level 4: hospitalization (typically used for detoxification of high risk patients, including pregnant patients, followed by a lower level of care).

ASAM has also established a category of "Special Populations" that includes elderly patients, healthcare professionals, or pregnant women (with and without children). The levels of care are typically elevated (often to Level 3) for these patients.

Additional information on monitoring during treatment, and individual treatment modalities, is available elsewhere in this monograph.

## Summary

In conclusion, there is no distinct line separating initial universal substance use screening from ongoing assessment and monitoring. It is important to maintain a reasonable index of suspicion even among those patients who have not been identified during initial screening and many of the tools are the same. Pregnancy offers an opportunity to identify patients with risky drinking or drug use and to provide appropriate treatment. A pregnant woman is motivated to do the best for her child and is more likely to disclose her use during pregnancy if she feels safe and understands that the health care provider truly has the best interests of her and her baby at heart. Nonetheless, women still face many obstacles including advanced addictive disease as well as the real fear of consequences from family, partners, the criminal justice system, and the child welfare system, which may prevent her from disclosing her use. Care must be taken to provide confidential, nonjudgmental medical care in order to build trust and improve pregnancy outcomes.

## References

1. Dowell D. H. T, Chou R. CDC guideline for prescribing opioids for chronic pain — United States, 2016. *MMWR Recomm Rep* 2016;65(No. RR-1):1–49. DOI: http://dx.doi.org/10.15585/mmwr.rr6501e1.

2. American Medical Association. *Using Prescription Drug Monitoring Programs*. Available from: www.ama-assn.org/content/using-prescription-drug-monitoring-programs.

3. National Association of Boards of Pharmacy. *PMP Interconnect*. Available from: https://nabp.pharmacy/initiatives/pmp-interconnect/.

4. Volkow N., McLellan T. Opioid abuse in chronic pain — misconceptions and mitigation strategies. *The New England Journal of Medicine*. 2016;374: 1253–63.

5. Ewing H. *A Practical Guide to Intervention in Health and Social Services, with Pregnant and Postpartum Addicts and Alcoholics*. Martinez, CA: The Born Free Project, Contra Costa County Department of Health Services; 1990.

6. Daetwyler C., Schindler B., Parran T. The clinical assessment of substance use disorders. *MedEdPORTAL* 2012. Available from: https://webcampus.drexelmed.edu/nida/module_1/default_FrameSet.html.

7. Guidice P. Cutaneous complications of intravenous drug use. *The British Journal of Dermatology*. 2004;150(1):1–10.

8. Fiebach N., Barker L., Burton J., Zieve P. *Principles of Ambulatory Medicine*. Philadelphia, PA: Lippincott Williams & Wilkins; 2007.

9. Bell J., Towers C. V., Hennessy M. D., et al. Detoxification from opiate drugs during pregnancy. *American Journal of Obstetrics and Gynecology*. 2016;215(3):374.e1–6.

10. Dennison S. Clonidine abuse among opioid addicts. *Psychiatric Quarterly*. 2001;72:191.

11. Shapiro B., Lynch K., Toochinda T., et al. Promethazine misuse among methadone maintenance patients and community-based injection drug users. *Journal of Addiction Medicine*. 2013;7(2):96–101.

12. Wilson J., Jungner G. *Principles and Practice of Screening for Disease*. Geneva: WHO; 1968.

Available from: www.who.int/bulletin/volumes/86/4/07-050112BP.pdf.

13. Patient Testing: Ethical Issues in Selection and Counseling. ACOG Committee Opinion No. 363. American College of Obstetricians and Gynecologists. *Obstetrics Gynecology*. 2007;109:1021–3.

14. Skipper G. E., Weinmann W., Thierauf A., et al. Ethyl glucuronide: A biomarker to identify alcohol use by health professionals recovering from substance use disorders. *Alcohol and Alcoholism*. 2004;39(5):445–9.

15. Mee-Lee D., Schulman G. D., Fishman M. J., et al. *The ASAM Criteria: Treatment Criteria for Addictive, Substance-Related, and Co-Occurring Conditions*, 3rd ed. Carson City, NV: The Change Companies; 2013.

# Co-occurring Mental Health Conditions in Pregnant Women with Opioid Use Disorders

Alexis S. Hammond and Margaret S. Chisolm

## Definitions

The brain is a highly complex organ from which the mind – with its diverse array of thoughts, feelings, and behaviors – emerges. Our mental life makes us uniquely human, and provides a richness of experience that is awe-inspiring. Our complex mental functioning can go awry at times, and when problems are idiosyncratic, sustained, pervasive, and/or interfere with functioning, they may rise to the level of a diagnosable mental health condition. Some of these disorders – like schizophrenia or bipolar affective disorder – can come out of the blue, unbidden, much like nonpsychiatric diseases such as cancer or diabetes. Other mental conditions begin only after exposure to an extraordinarily adverse event or – in someone with personality vulnerabilities – to more routine stressful events. Some mental conditions are more behavioral in nature, such as eating disorders (ED), sexual disorders (e.g., pedophilia, voyeurism) and substance use disorders (SUD), which typically begin with an initial choice to engage in the behavior, followed by a pleasurable effect that leads to the behavior happening repeatedly as the drive becomes stronger and the choice more difficult to resist [1]. Women with opioid use disorders (OUD) in pregnancy are – by definition – suffering from at least one mental health condition. However, the likelihood that they have another co-occurring disorder is quite high.

## Incidence/Epidemiology

Pregnant and postpartum women – compared to non-pregnant women – seem to have significantly lower rates of most mental health conditions, including SUD. (The main exception is found among postpartum women who may have significantly higher rates of major depressive disorder [MDD]) [2]. Suggested risk factors for increased rates of mental health conditions among pregnant and postpartum women include SUD, personal history of other mental illness, young adult age, lack of social support, a negative attitude toward pregnancy, current or previous pregnancy complications, stressors, and a history of trauma [2–6].

How do prevalence rates of mental health conditions compare between pregnant women with SUD and those without SUD? Not surprisingly, pregnant women with SUD tend to have higher rates of comorbid mental health conditions than pregnant women without SUD. For example, one study reported women with an SUD had 3 times the odds of having a psychiatric illness than women without SUD [7]. Opioid-dependent pregnant women are at increased risk for personality disorders, post-traumatic stress disorder (PTSD), anxiety, depression, and bipolar affective disorder [8].

A large, multisite study of opioid-dependent pregnant women found 65 percent who endorsed symptoms consistent with one or more mental health condition (49 percent mood disorder; 40 percent anxiety disorder). Compared to the opioid-dependent women without psychiatric symptoms, they had more impairment on the Addiction Severity Scale, especially in the domains of Family/Social Functioning, and Psychological Functioning. Those who reported symptoms of MDD, dysthymia, hypomania, generalized anxiety disorder (GAD), PTSD and suicidality had significantly higher scores in substance use severity [9].

These and other epidemiologic findings suggesting high prevalence of mental health conditions among pregnant/postpartum women with SUD highlight the importance of screening for such disorders in this population. Pregnant women are an especially important population to screen for these illnesses, as they not only affect the health of the mother, but also can adversely impact the pregnancy and the baby. Additionally, due to the effects of psychiatric symptoms on substance use (and vice versa) and psychosocial functioning, evaluation and effective treatment should be a routine part of managing pregnant women with SUD.

## Principals of Assessment and Treatment

Although psychiatrists are the only physicians trained exclusively in the evaluation and treatment of disordered thoughts, feelings, and behaviors, patients with mental health concerns usually seek and receive treatment from nonpsychiatric primary care providers. The American Psychiatric Association's *Diagnostic and Statistical Manual of Mental Disorders (DSM)* provides a common language by which clinicians – regardless of specialty training – and researchers can more reliably diagnose patients, and the *DSM* has led to some modest advancements in treatment. However, the *DSM* must not be the sole basis of a patient's evaluation. The *DSM* is meant only "to *assist* trained clinicians in the diagnosis of their patients' mental disorders *as part of* a case formulation assessment [emphasis ours] that leads to a fully informed treatment plan for each individual." [10] Clinicians are meant to not rely on the *DSM's* helpful checklist of signs and symptoms as the sole means to formulate a patient's condition. Instead clinicians are advised to use the *DSM* as just one part of the assessment and to take into consideration the multiple and complex aspects of each individual who comes to them for help [11].

For the primary care clinician who is first evaluating a pregnant woman with OUD or co-occurring mental health conditions, the following streamlined approach (Box 4.1) is recommended.

## Behavioral Treatments and Mental Hygiene

Women who use opioids in pregnancy and also have co-occurring mental health conditions need specialized services designed to optimize treatment outcomes for both their opioid use and their co-occurring disorders. Normal mental life relies on healthy biological *and* psychological functioning, which can be influenced by a variety of factors. When normal mental functioning goes awry, treatments based in the sciences of biology and psychology – and even sociology – are often necessary. For example, both biological treatments – such as methadone, buprenorphine, naltrexone – and psychological treatments – such as motivational interviewing, cognitive behavioral therapy, contingency management – are effective for OUD, and are often most effective in combination.

When opioid-using pregnant women have co-occurring mental health conditions, both pharmacologic and behavioral treatments – along with social supports – are usually necessary for successful outcomes. In addition to prescribing medications to remedy any obvious mental diseases like manias or severe depressions, clinicians need to engage patients in individual talk therapy. One goal of psychotherapy is to help women make sense of the losses they have encountered because of their opioid use and other mental health condition(s) and to offer hope that they can overcome these and any future challenges. Clinicians can also help women better understand their individual personalities, help them set goals, and guide them through all of life's provocations, steering a steady course toward wellness. Couples and family therapy can also be helpful, even for patients with brain-based diseases like schizophrenia and manic depressive illness. It is helpful to talk directly with patients and their families about how pharmacologic and behavioral treatments can be enhanced by social supports based in the domains of family, community, education, and employment. For example, less expressed emotion in families improves treatment outcomes in schizophrenia [12] and regular religious service attendance can lower the risk of suicide [13].

## Introduction to Medication in Pregnancy

When evaluation of an opioid-dependent pregnant woman indicates that pharmacologic treatment is appropriate (likely in addition to psychotherapy), the available options must be weighed for each individual patient and situation. We will review what is currently known about the use of psychotropic medications in pregnancy, though this is not an exhaustive list including all risks and benefits (please see [14] for a more detailed discussion). When deciding whether to prescribe a psychotropic medication to a pregnant woman, there are several key factors to consider (Figure 4.1). Not only should the risks and benefits of treating the mother be considered, but one must also contemplate the potential risk of medication exposure to the fetus. The risks of untreated illness for the mother and fetus should also be taken into account, as some conditions have life-threatening consequences when untreated, including suicide, and can also serve as an exposure to the fetus that can affect subsequent development of the child.

**Box 4.1**

1. Gather a family history of psychiatric illness including depression, mania, schizophrenia, attempted/completed suicides, and attention problems.
2. Inquire about any childhood illnesses and behavioral symptoms (e.g., fire setting, animal cruelty, fighting, truancy). Ask about potential attention disorder symptoms (e.g., inattention, hyperactivity, impulsivity) and any special education requirements.
3. Take an educational and occupational history.
4. Obtain a sexual history (including any sexual abuse) and marital/relationship history (e.g., partner substance use, supportiveness, interpersonal violence). Ask where she is currently living and any recent history of homelessness. Also inquire about religious affiliations.
5. Document legal history and, if available, conduct an online state judiciary case search (each state maintains its own website for which one can search online).
6. Obtain a detailed substance use history, including any tobacco, alcohol, marijuana, and cocaine use, as well as use of other illicit drugs (e.g., LSD, MDMA, PCP, methamphetamine, synthetic marijuana, solvents, inhalants, caffeine) and prescription drug abuse (e.g., amphetamines, benzodiazepines). For each drug, include route (e.g., intranasal, intravenous, inhalation), age at first use, age at first daily use, current use and duration, maximum use, last use, longest abstinence (date/length/context), and withdrawal symptoms. Also include any prior substance abuse treatment, including medically supervised withdrawal, rehabilitation programs and pharmacologic treatment (e.g., methadone, buprenorphine, disulfiram, naltrexone).
7. Document other medical and surgical history, outpatient providers (primary care provider, psychiatrist, therapist, case manager), and the patient's current medications and drug allergies.
8. A complete review of systems is needed.
9. Clarify any past history of mental health concerns, identifying time of first onset (e.g., childhood), without regard to treatment-seeking. Symptoms during periods of abstinence from opioids and/or other substances should be noted. Include all suicide attempts with age, description of method, circumstances, and any medical consequences to best understand both the intent and potential lethality of each attempt. Include all psychotropic medication trials with dose, duration, side effects, and efficacy.
10. Outline a description of the events leading to the current presentation, including a detailed history of substance use, recurrence of symptoms, medication nonadherence, and life stressors. Again, inquire about the temporal relationship between opioid and/or other substance use and any change in the patient's thoughts, feelings, and behaviors.
11. Conduct a thorough mental status examination, including assessments of affect (mood, sleep, appetite, energy, concentration, and view of self/future (including suicidal thoughts, plans, intentions)), hallucinations, delusions, orientation, and memory.
12. Conduct a thorough physical examination.
13. Obtain laboratory testing including toxicology screens.
14. Electrocardiogram for QT interval monitoring may be indicated. This is especially important for patients who are receiving or may receive methadone-assisted treatment, which is associated with prolongation of the QT interval and possible cardiac arrhythmia (Torsade des Pointes).

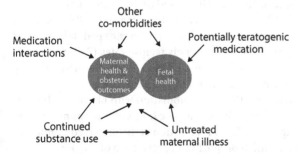

**Figure 4.1** General factors to consider when forming a treatment plan for a pregnant woman with OUD, and their potential effects on the health of the mother and fetus

## Diagnosis-Specific Management

Given the risks that maternal mental health conditions pose for both mother and child, restoring a pregnant woman to mental health is a high priority. Each woman's past psychiatric history, severity of symptoms, medication response and wishes regarding pharmacologic treatment during pregnancy must be explored prior to developing an individualized treatment plan [14]. Each plan should include a combination of pharmacologic and behavioral treatment strategies.

# Attention Deficit Hyperactivity Disorder (ADHD)

The prevalence of ADHD is greater among individuals with substance use – including opioid-using women – than in the general population. At its core, ADHD is a condition in which an individual is less able to inhibit impulses – to move, to act, to pay attention to less salient stimuli, resulting in the classic ADHD triad of hyperactivity, impulsivity, and inattention. Pharmacologic treatments include stimulant (e.g., methylphenidate, dextroamphetamine) and nonstimulant (atomoxetine, guanfacine) medications. The best studied of these in pregnancy are methylphenidate and atomoxetine [15–18]. Pharmacologic treatments for ADHD are unlikely to be initiated during pregnancy, as the benefits of medication use during pregnancy – given that ADHD is rarely a life-threatening condition – are unlikely to outweigh the risks. Also, because most stimulant medications can be misused and carry with them the risk of addiction, these are especially unlikely to be initiated in opioid-using women during pregnancy. However, pharmacologic treatments are just one component of ADHD care. Behavioral treatments are critically important in the long-term treatment of these disorders, as well. Although a discussion of these is beyond the scope of this review, the interested reader is referred to several recent reviews on this topic [19, 20].

# Major Depressive Disorder (MDD)

Hallmark symptoms of MDD include pervasive and sustained changes in mood – irritability and/or sadness – and a change in one's outlook toward self or the future, manifest often as guilt or hopelessness. An episode of MDD may also be heralded by a change in one's sleep, appetite, concentration, energy level, ability to experience pleasure, and/or social engagement. Careful screening for MDD among women of reproductive age is imperative, as this condition is relatively common during pregnancy with a prevalence of about 8–13 percent, and depressive symptoms during pregnancy have been associated with poor outcomes such as low birth weight and preterm birth [21]. Depression has also been found to be associated with risk factors that would affect pregnancy outcomes such as substance use (including smoking), hypertension, gestational diabetes, and preeclampsia [21]. Among pregnant women with SUD, about 40–73 percent have comorbid depression and about 50 percent have postpartum depression 6 weeks after delivery [22]. Studies of pregnant women

with OUD who were maintained on methadone and had co-occurring depression suggest poor outcomes, such as lower clinic attendance, and more drug-positive urine samples [22] (Figure 4.1).

The most commonly studied class of antidepressant medication includes selective serotonin reuptake inhibitors (SSRIs), which have been found to be safe in pregnancy among most studies [23–26]. Similarly, most studies have not associated use of tricyclic antidepressants (TCA) [27–30], or other antidepressants [31, 32] with major malformations. There are several conditions that have been discussed in relation to newborns who were exposed to antidepressants *in utero*, including poor neonatal adaptation syndrome, persistent pulmonary hypertension of the newborn, and autism spectrum disorder. Most of the studies showing these effects are retrospective, introducing recall bias, and suffer from poor design, not controlling for the effects of the maternal mental illness itself [14, 33].

In addition to medication, there are particular modalities of psychotherapy that are helpful for MDD. When considering using psychotherapy alone, or in combination with medication, severity of illness and efficacy of the particular psychotherapy should be considered. A particular modality with known efficacy for both MDD and SUD is cognitive-behavioral therapy (CBT). CBT for depression in pregnancy has been found to be effective, and the combination of CBT and medication for depression during pregnancy and the postpartum period has been found to be more helpful than medication alone or CBT alone [34].

# Bipolar Affective Disorder (BPAD)

Symptoms of BPAD included mood lability, with irritability, anger or euphoric/expansive mood, impulsivity, lack of need for sleep, pressured speech, high self-attitude and increased goal-directed activity. There is a high rate of disease recurrence (81–85.5 percent) among pregnant women who stopped taking their mood stabilizers versus relapse rates (29–37 percent) of women who maintained their pharmacotherapy during pregnancy [35, 36]. The use of CBT is effective for BPAD in combination with pharmacotherapy, but there is little evidence for its efficacy as monotherapy [34]. Thus, medication is the preferred method of treatment of BPAD and prevention of relapse.

Mood stabilizers are commonly used for treatment of BPAD. Lamotrigine is an effective and relatively safe [37] medication for treatment of BPAD, though levels may need to be followed for dose adjustments during pregnancy [38]. Use of valproic acid and carbamazepine during pregnancy is not generally recommended due to safety concerns for the fetus [39]. Lithium use during pregnancy has been associated with an increased risk of the serious, but very rare, congenital heart defect known as Ebstein's anomaly [40]. Again, the severity of maternal illness should be considered when weighing the risks of taking lithium, and, if used, blood levels should be followed, as higher doses may be required, with a reduction or discontinuation at the time of labor to avoid toxicity [14]. Neuroleptic medications with indications for BPAD such as lurasidone have also been used in pregnancy and are discussed in the section on schizophrenia.

## Delirium and Dementia

A temporarily altered level of consciousness is often a desired effect of substance use, and is often associated with a temporary but global decline in cognitive functioning called delirium. Delirium can result from substance use/intoxication, as well as withdrawal from certain substances (alcohol, benzodiazepines). Additionally, it can be caused by systemic or brain infections, and other – often very serious – medical causes. In order to treat delirium, the specific etiology must first be identified. For some causes of delirium (such as hallucinogen-induced delirium), the primary treatment is time and supportive therapy. For other causes such as alcohol withdrawal delirium (also known as delirium tremens), the treatment would involve a benzodiazepine or other medication taper. Because of the severe and potentially life-threatening nature of delirium, pregnancy is usually not a contraindication for treatment.

Chronic substance use can also result in a global decline of cognitive functioning, but – unlike with delirium – this decline is usually permanent and not accompanied by a normal level of consciousness. Psychiatrists describe this permanent decline as dementia, and it is usually caused by chronic use of extremely neurotoxic substances such as alcohol or inhalants. Unfortunately, treatment for dementia is largely supportive.

## Insomnia

Sleep during pregnancy – especially the third trimester – is often elusive, due to fetal movement, gastroesophageal reflux and other physical changes. Over 90 percent of pregnant women report using over-the-counter antihistamines (e.g., diphenhydramine, doxylamine, hydroxyzine) to help with insomnia [41]. Although a systematic review of antihistamines and birth defects described an association between fetal antihistamine exposure and congenital malformations, the studies reviewed had serious methodological limitations [42]. Another review identified only one study on this topic and it showed no association between fetal antihistamine exposure and congenital malformations [43].

Prescription sleep aids are also used in pregnancy, although less commonly than the over-the-counter medications. Because benzodiazepines are highly addictive and are often used for euphoric effect in combination with opioids, they are usually contraindicated in women with OUD. In addition, benzodiazepine use has been associated with multiple adverse neonatal outcomes including low APGAR scores, poor feeding, and – in some studies – cleft palate defects [44, 45]. Thus, the use of benzodiazepines for insomnia in this population is minimal. Benzodiazepine-like sleep agents (eszopiclone, ramelteon, and zolpidem) have not been associated with major organ malformations [43], but longer-term (greater than 90 days) zolpidem use has been associated with low birth weight, preterm birth and cesarean delivery [46]. CBT for insomnia is considered to be the first-line treatment and would be especially appropriate during pregnancy [47, 48].

## Anxiety Disorders

Because anxiety disorders – particularly PTSD – are discussed elsewhere in this volume, only a few important points will be briefly mentioned here. Rates of anxiety disorders among pregnant women with SUD may be quite high. One study found a prevalence of 43 percent for GAD, 28 percent for panic disorder, 26 percent for agoraphobia, 22 percent for social phobia/social anxiety, and 18 percent for PTSD [49]. Opioid-dependent pregnant women with anxiety are more likely to stop treatment compared to those without anxiety [22].

CBT is a first-line treatment for anxiety, and thus is a particularly helpful tool to use in pregnant women to avoid unnecessary exposure to the fetus with medication. For moderate to severe cases, the addition of an SSRI is often needed, and proves effective [35]. Other techniques, such as supportive and psychodynamic therapies, exercise and relaxation can be tried, with a goal being to provide patients with healthy coping skills to avoid self-medication and relapse on illicit drugs [50]. As mentioned, benzodiazepines should be avoided in this population. Gabapentin has been used off-label for treatment of anxiety. While multiple studies have not found an increased risk of major malformations in infants exposed to gabapentin *in utero* [51, 52], higher rates of poor outcomes with gabapentin use have been noted including low birth weight, preterm birth and a longer stay in intensive care [53]. Pregabalin is another medication that has been used off-label for treatment of anxiety, and has not been found to increase risk of malformations. Another option is buspirone, which has not been found to be teratogenic in animal studies, though no studies in humans have been performed [14].

## Eating Disorders (ED)

These disorders are more common among women with SUD (17–46 percent) than the general population (3 percent) [54, 55], though they are often not screened for, or treated. In particular, bulimic behavior is more common in this population than restricting behaviors. Use of various substances by women with ED may be explained by the substances' potential to assist with weight loss, manage negative affect, and treat physical symptoms [55]. Because ED come with their own serious complications, a co-occurring SUD can lead to higher rates of medical complications and illness relapse.

About 1 percent of all pregnant women have a prior diagnosis of anorexia nervosa and bulimia nervosa. Active ED during pregnancy have been associated with multiple adverse outcomes for the mother baby dyad including nutritional deficiencies, intrauterine growth retardation, cesarean delivery, fetal neural tube defects, negative feelings toward pregnancy, postpartum depression, and infant developmental delay [56].

There is a need for further study on treatments of co-occurring ED and SUD, but the current view is to treat both disorders concurrently, using a multi-disciplinary approach so that symptoms of one illness do not interfere with recovery from the other [54, 55]. Management of the pregnant woman with an eating disorder is identical to that of a nonpregnant woman, with the addition of an obstetrician to the treatment team [56]. Ensuring medical stability is paramount, which may require hospitalization [54]. Once medically stable, behavior therapy alone has been found to be more effective than CBT for bulimia nervosa. Motivational interviewing is particularly helpful for the pregnant woman with an eating disorder, as most recognize the importance of healthy eating for the wellbeing of the fetus. SSRIs may provide some benefit for ED, especially bulimia, as they are more helpful in women of normal weight [50, 55, 56].

## Schizophrenia

This condition is relatively rare among pregnant women with SUD, with a prevalence that appears similar to the general population (1–2 percent) [22]. Symptoms include both positive symptoms (hallucinations, delusions, thought disorder) and negative symptoms (withdrawal, anhedonia, social withdrawal). Schizophrenia's negative symptoms may explain the low rates of this condition among women who use substances, as volition is so reduced. Antipsychotic medications, also known as neuroleptics, are the mainstay of treatment for this condition, in addition to psychosocial treatments for the patient and family. These medications have generally been found to be safe in pregnancy, and the benefits likely outweigh the risk of untreated serious mental illness. Because of the association between antipsychotics – particularly second-generation antipsychotics (e.g., aripiprazole, quetiapine) – and metabolic dysregulation, including gestational diabetes, women taking these medications should have routine monitoring of fetal size in late pregnancy. Women taking first-generation antipsychotic medications (e.g., haloperidol, thioridazine) should be monitored for anti-cholinergic effects such as orthostatic hypotension [14].

## Conclusions

Like other major medical conditions, mental health conditions that co-occur among pregnant women with OUD need to be diagnosed and treated for the overall health and well-being of mothers – including recovery from OUD – and their children. This chapter provides a broad overview for nonpsychiatrists to help with mental health assessment, including recognition of symptomatology, and general treatment guidelines in pregnancy. However, complicated cases may benefit from consultation with, and/or evaluation by psychiatrists, with a sustained team approach involving the patient and her family.

## References

1. McHugh P. R. and Slavney P. R. *The Perspectives of Psychiatry*. Baltimore: JHU Press; 2011.

2. Vesga-Lopez O., Blanco C., Keyes K., et al. Psychiatric disorders in pregnant and postpartum women in the United States. *Arch Gen Psychiatry* 2008; 65:805–15.

3. Leigh B. and Milgrom J. Risk factors for antenatal depression, postnatal depression and parenting stress. *BMC Psychiatry* 2008; 8:24.

4. Marcus S. M. and Heringhausen J. E. Depression in childbearing women: When depression complicates pregnancy. *Prim Care: Clin Office Practice* 2009; 36:151–65.

5. Norhayati M., Hazlina N. N., Asrenee A., Emilin W. W. Magnitude and risk factors for postpartum symptoms: A literature review. *J Affect Disord* 2015; 175:34–52.

6. Biaggi A., Conroy S., Pawlby S., Pariante C. M. Identifying the women at risk of antenatal anxiety and depression: A systematic review. *J Affect Disord* 2016; 191:62–77.

7. Kennare R., Heard A., Chan A. Substance use during pregnancy: Risk factors and obstetric and perinatal outcomes in South Australia. *Austral New Zeal J Obstet Gynaecol* 2005; 45:220–5.

8. Krans E. E., Cochran G., Bogen D. L. Caring for opioid-dependent pregnant women: Prenatal and postpartum care considerations. *Clin Obstet Gynecol* 2015; 58:370–9.

9. Benningfield M. M., Arria A. M., Kaltenbach K., et al. Co-occurring psychiatric symptoms are associated with increased psychological, social, and medical impairment in opioid dependent pregnant women. *Am J Addict* 2010; 19:416–21.

10. American Psychiatric Association. Use of the Manual. In: American Psychiatric Association, editors. *Diagnostic and Statistical Manual of Mental Disorders.* Arlington http://dx.doi.org/10.1176/appi .books.9780890425596.UseofDSM5; 2013. p. 19.

11. Chisolm M. S. and Lyketsos C. G. *Systematic Psychiatric Evaluation: A Step-by-Step Guide to Applying the Perspectives of Psychiatry.* Baltimore: JHU Press; 2012.

12. Kavanagh D. J. Recent developments in expressed emotion and schizophrenia. *Br J Psychiatry* 1992; 160:601–20.

13. VanderWeele T. J., Li S., Tsai A. C., Kawachi I. Association between religious service attendance and lower suicide rates among US women. *JAMA Psychiatry* 2016; 73:845–51.

14. Chisolm M. S. and Payne J. L. Management of psychotropic drugs during pregnancy. *BMJ* 2016; 532:h5918.

15. Bolea-Alamanac B. M., Green A., Verma G., Maxwell P., Davies S. J. Methylphenidate use in pregnancy and lactation: A systematic review of evidence. *Br J Clin Pharmacol* 2014; 77:96–101.

16. Dadashova R. and Silverstone P. H. Off-label use of atomoxetine in adults: Is it safe? *Ment Illn* 2012; 4:e19.

17. Hærvig K. B., Mortensen L. H., Hansen A. V., Strandberg-Larsen K. Use of ADHD medication during pregnancy from 1999 to 2010: A Danish register-based study. *Pharmacoepidemiol Drug Saf* 2014; 23:526–33.

18. Pottegård A., Hallas J., Andersen J. T., et al. First-trimester exposure to methylphenidate: A population-based cohort study. *J Clin Psychiatry* 2014; 75:88–93.

19. Chandler M. Psychotherapy for adult attention deficit/hyperactivity disorder: A comparison with cognitive behaviour therapy. *J Psychiatr Ment Health Nurs* 2013; 20:814–20.

20. Manos M. J. Psychosocial therapy in the treatment of adults with attention-deficit/hyperactivity disorder. *Postgrad Med* 2013; 125:51–64.

21. Grote N. K., Bridge J. A., Gavin A. R., et al. A meta-analysis of depression during pregnancy and the risk of preterm birth, low birth weight, and intrauterine growth restriction. *Arch Gen Psychiatry* 2010; 67:1012–24.

22. Jones H. Caring for the Dually Diagnosed Patient. In: Hendrée Jones and Karol Kaltenbach, editors. *Treating Women with Substance use Disorders during Pregnancy: A Comprehensive Approach to Caring for Mother and Child.* New York: Oxford University Press; 2013. p. 111–28.

23. Addis A. and Koren G. Safety of fluoxetine during the first trimester of pregnancy: A meta-analytical review of epidemiological studies. *Psychol Med* 2000; 30:89–94.

24. Einarson T. R. and Einarson A. Newer antidepressants in pregnancy and rates of major malformations: A meta-analysis of prospective comparative studies. *Pharmacoepidemiol Drug Saf* 2005; 14:823–7.

25. O'Brien L., Einarson T. R., Sarkar M., Einarson A., Koren G. Does paroxetine cause cardiac malformations? *J Obstet Gynaecol Can* 2008; 30:696–701.

26. Rahimi R., Nikfar S., Abdollahi M. Pregnancy outcomes following exposure to serotonin reuptake inhibitors: A meta-analysis of clinical trials. *Reprod Toxicol* 2006; 22:571–5.

27. Davis R. L., Rubanowice D., McPhillips H., et al. Risks of congenital malformations and perinatal events among infants exposed to antidepressant medications during pregnancy. *Pharmacoepidemiol Drug Saf* 2007; 16:1086–94.

28. Nulman I., Rovet J., Stewart D. E., et al. Neurodevelopment of children exposed in utero to antidepressant drugs. *N Engl J Med* 1997; 336:258–62.

29. Simon G. E., Cunningham M. L., Davis R. L. Outcomes of prenatal antidepressant exposure. *Am J Psychiatry* 2002; 159:2055–61.

30. Ramos E., St-Andre M., Rey E., Oraichi D., Berard A. Duration of antidepressant use during pregnancy and risk of major congenital malformations. *Br J Psychiatry* 2008; 192:344–50.

31. Byatt N., Deligiannidis K. M., Freeman M. P. Antidepressant use in pregnancy: A critical review focused on risks and controversies. *Acta Psychiatr Scand* 2013; 127:94–114.

32. Yonkers K. A., Blackwell K. A., Glover J., Forray A. Antidepressant use in pregnant and postpartum women. *Annu Rev Clin Psychol* 2014; 10:369–92.

33. Chambers C. D., Hernandez-Diaz S., Van Marter L. J., et al. Selective serotonin-reuptake inhibitors and risk of persistent pulmonary hypertension of the newborn. *N Engl J Med* 2006; 354:579–87.

34. Hofmann S. G., Asnaani A., Vonk I. J., Sawyer A. T., Fang A. The efficacy of cognitive behavioral therapy: A review of meta-analyses. *Cogn TherRes* 2012; 36:427–40.

35. Viguera A. C., Nonacs R., Cohen L. S., et al. Risk of recurrence of bipolar disorder in pregnant and nonpregnant women after discontinuing lithium maintenance. *Am J Psychiatry* 2000; 157:179–84.

36. Viguera A. C., Whitfield T., Baldessarini R. J., et al. Risk of recurrence in women with bipolar disorder during pregnancy: Prospective study of mood stabilizer discontinuation. *Am J Psychiatry* 2007; 164:1817–24.

37. Dolk H., Jentink J., Loane M., Morris J., de Jong-van den Berg L. T., EUROCAT Antiepileptic Drug Working Group. Does lamotrigine use in pregnancy increase orofacial cleft risk relative to other malformations? *Neurology* 2008; 71:714–22.

38. Clark C. T., Klein A. M., Perel J. M., Helsel J., Wisner K. L. Lamotrigine dosing for pregnant patients with bipolar disorder. *Am J Psychiatry* 2013; 170:1240–7.

39. Pearlstein T. Use of psychotropic medication during pregnancy and the postpartum period. *Womens Health* 2013; 9:605–15.

40. Cohen L. S., Friedman J., Jefferson J. W., Johnson E. M., Weiner M. L. A reevaluation of risk of in utero exposure to lithium. *JAMA* 1994; 271:146–50.

41. Black R. A. and Hill D. A. Over-the-counter medications in pregnancy. *Am Fam Physician* 2003; 67:2517–24.

42. Gilboa S. M., Ailes E. C., Rai R. P., Anderson J. A., Honein M. A. Antihistamines and birth defects: A systematic review of the literature. *Expert Opin Drug Saf* 2014; 13:1667–98.

43. Okun M. L., Ebert R., Saini B. A review of sleep-promoting medications used in pregnancy. *Obstet Gynecol* 2015; 212:428–41.

44. Iqbal M. M., Sobhan T., Ryals T. Effects of commonly used benzodiazepines on the fetus, the neonate, and the nursing infant. *Psychiatr Serv* 2002; 53:39–49.

45. Lin A. E., Peller A. J., Westgate M., et al. Clonazepam use in pregnancy and the risk of malformations. *Birth Defects Res Part A: Clin Mol Teratol* 2004; 70:534–6.

46. Wang L., Lin H., Lin C., Chen Y. Increased risk of adverse pregnancy outcomes in women receiving zolpidem during pregnancy. *Clin Pharmacol Ther* 2010; 88:369–74.

47. Smith M. T., Huang M. I., Manber R. Cognitive behavior therapy for chronic insomnia occurring within the context of medical and psychiatric disorders. *Clin Psychol Rev* 2005; 25:559–92.

48. Taylor D. J. and Pruiksma K. E. Cognitive and behavioural therapy for insomnia (CBT-I) in psychiatric populations: A systematic review. *Int Rev Psychiatry* 2014; 26:205–13.

49. Martin P. R., Arria A. M., Fischer G., et al. Psychopharmacologic management of opioid-dependent women during pregnancy. *Am J Addict* 2009; 18:148–56.

50. Zweben J. Special Issues in Treatment: Women. In: Richard Ries, Shannon Miller, David Fiellin and Richard Saitz, editors. *The ASAM Principles of Addiction Medicine*, Fifth Edition. Hong Kong: Wolters Kluwer Health; 2014. p. 524–34.

51. Holmes L. B. and Hernandez-Diaz S. Newer anticonvulsants: Lamotrigine, topiramate and gabapentin. *Birth Defects Res Part A: Clin Mol Teratol* 2012; 94:599–606.

52. Mølgaard-Nielsen D. and Hviid A. Newer-generation antiepileptic drugs and the risk of major birth defects. *JAMA* 2011; 305:1996–2002.

53. Fujii H., Goel A., Bernard N., et al. Pregnancy outcomes following gabapentin use: Results of a prospective comparative cohort study. *Neurology* 2013; 80:1565–70.

54. Harrop E. N. and Marlatt G. A. The comorbidity of substance use disorders and eating disorders in women: Prevalence, etiology, and treatment. *Addict Behav* 2010; 35:392–8.

55. Gregorowski C., Seedat S., Jordaan G. P. A clinical approach to the assessment and management of co-morbid eating disorders and substance use disorders. *BMC Psychiatry* 2013; 13:1.

56. Cardwell M. S. Eating disorders during pregnancy. *Obstet Gynecol Surv* 2013; 68:312–23.

# 5

# Trauma and Posttraumatic Stress Disorder in Women with Opioid-Use Disorder in Pregnancy

Soraya Asadi

Joanne is a 34-year-old female veteran with longstanding heroin use who presents for prenatal care in the late first trimester. Several years ago, Joanne became homeless and was sexually assaulted. Subsequent to this event, she decided to sleep nightly in a garbage dumpster to increase her sense of security. Several months later when the dumpster was emptied into a garbage collection truck, Joanne's arm was severely injured in the truck's compactor.

With medication-assisted treatment for opioid-use disorder, Joanne is eventually able to stop using heroin in her second trimester as evidenced by repeated negative urine drug screens. She goes on to have a full-term vaginal delivery complicated by a second-degree perineal tear. Shortly thereafter staff members from child protective services arrive after being contacted by a nurse who has read "opioid-use disorder" in Joanne's medical record but who is otherwise unfamiliar with Joanne's case. It takes a few hours for Joanne's current treatment status to be clarified. However, for the rest of her hospital stay Joanne is emotionally distressed and so kept under constant surveillance of the area near the pediatric intensive care unit.

Pregnant women who have histories of trauma and opioid use frequently present to the medical setting with unique biopsychosocial needs. Social stigmatization related to both trauma and addiction can also present a major barrier to improved health outcomes. In recent decades, identification of gender-linked trauma has become recognized as an important component in the integrated and interdisciplinary care of women with addiction [1]. This chapter provides an overview of current prevalence, screening and assessment approaches, and effective clinical practices for gender-linked trauma and posttraumatic stress disorder (PTSD) as they relate to pregnant women with opioid-use disorder.

Examples of trauma that disproportionately affect women include childhood sexual abuse, intimate partner violence, sexual trauma occurring in the context of military service, and traumatic childbirth. A potential consequence of gender-linked trauma PTSD is a mental health disorder that can arise from trauma related to a single event, a series of repeated or resultant events, or a chronic condition. Trauma meeting diagnostic criteria for PTSD requires exposure to actual or threatened death, serious injury, or sexual violence, and is inclusive of such events whether they are experienced directly or indirectly. PTSD is also defined by four cluster symptoms: intrusive reexperiencing of the event, avoidance of stimuli associated with the event, persistent negative alterations in cognition and mood, and alterations in arousal and reactivity [2].

PTSD is a disorder that disproportionately affects women. Prevalence estimates of lifetime PTSD from large national surveys consistently indicate that PTSD is more common in women than men in the general population [3, 4]. It has been postulated that higher lifetime prevalence of PTSD in women may partially relate to gender differences in hormonal responses to stress as well as to higher lifetime rates of sexual trauma among women as compared to men. Traumatic injury during pregnancy is most commonly associated with motor vehicle crashes and intimate partner violence but suicide, homicide, falls, burns, accidental poisoning, penetrating trauma, and toxic exposure also contribute to injury during pregnancy [5].

In both pregnant and postpartum women, a history of such stressful or traumatic life events has been found to be significantly associated with higher risk of comorbid psychiatric disorders [6]. Current research suggests that PTSD is higher in the perinatal population and that higher rates of detachment, loss of interest, anger and irritability, trouble sleeping, and nightmares

| Intrusive reexperiencing | Avoidance | Cognition and mood | Arousal and reactivity |
|---|---|---|---|
| Recurrent, involuntary memories<br>Nightmares<br>Flashbacks<br>Losing awareness of present time and place (dissociation)<br>Intense distress when triggered by reminders of event (can include infant) | Avoidance of trauma-related emotions or thoughts<br>Avoidance of trauma-related stimuli (may include infant in case of perinatal trauma) | Inability to recall key features of the event (can manifest as dissociative amnesia during the exam or during childbirth)<br>Diminished interest in activities<br>Persistent negative beliefs about oneself, others, or the world ("I'm a bad mother")<br>Distorted thoughts about the cause/consequences of the event or self-blame<br>Detachment or estrangement from others (can include infant)<br>Persistent negative emotional state or inability to experience positive emotions | Sleep difficulty<br>Self-destructive behaviors<br>Outbursts of irritability or anger<br>Increased startle response<br>Difficulty with concentration<br>Hypervigilance (can manifest in overly protective stance towards infant) |

**Figure 5.1** Sample cluster symptoms of PTSD in the perinatal period

occur in this population [7]. Pregnant women with a diagnosis of PTSD have also been found to have higher risk for perinatal complications such as ectopic pregnancy, spontaneous abortion, hyperemesis, preterm contractions, excessive fetal growth [8], and preterm birth [9]. Additionally, anticipatory anxiety and lived experiences related to pregnancy, labor, and childrearing have also been suggested as potential causal pathways for trauma-related symptoms. In women with low partner support and unplanned pregnancy, higher prevalence rates of PTSD have been found in the postpartum period [10]. Maternal PTSD during pregnancy and associated changes in stress hormones may also have as yet unknown potential epigenetic and developmental consequences in regards to outcomes in offspring [11].

When opioid-use disorder intersects with trauma exposure, a woman's ability to protect herself, access support, negotiate safe sex practices, or avoid sharing drug-use equipment may be limited. A bidirectional relationship between substance use and trauma has been qualitatively described in the literature as continuing during the course of pregnancy [12]. Past-year prevalence of PTSD in women has been found to be significantly associated with both nonmedical opioid-use and opioid-use disorder [13], and female gender has been found to be a risk factor for traumatic event reexposure among injection drug users [14]. Pregnancy or the presence of other children in the home may promote maintenance of an abusive relationship with a drug-using partner for emotional or financial reasons. Trauma sequelae such as physical injury or pain may lead to exposure to prescribed or illicit opiates, and child abuse potential may also increase [15, 16].

Current studies from multiple disciplinary fields suggest that gendered experiences of trauma and substance use disorder may be linked to interrelated biomedical, environmental, health systems, and sexual/reproductive factors. These intersecting areas of research are summarized in Figure 5.2.

However, while a paradigm shift toward transdisciplinarity and integration has increasingly evolved in the field of research [17], trauma-specific services for women with substance use disorders remain limited in the addiction services sector [18]. This finding presents an opportunity for the broader medical community to adopt services that are trauma-informed. By definition, trauma-informed care indirectly acknowledges the impact of trauma at the individual and societal levels and focuses on the general engagement and support of women with trauma histories. Training resources and self-assessment tools for organizations that wish to become trauma-informed can be found in the public domain [19].

A trauma-informed approach promotes awareness and recognition of trauma-related symptoms. Research suggests that in clinical interactions with pregnant women, treatment providers often do not elicit histories of trauma-related symptoms or PTSD [20, 21]. It is unclear whether this relates to limited appointment time, lack of training, or fears that exploring the trauma may precipitate increased substance use. However, it appears that trauma-related symptoms can be concomitantly identified and addressed with substance use disorders without precipitating adverse events [22]. Additionally, as trauma-related symptoms such as sleep disturbance can overlap with other mental health disorders or be a product of pregnancy itself,

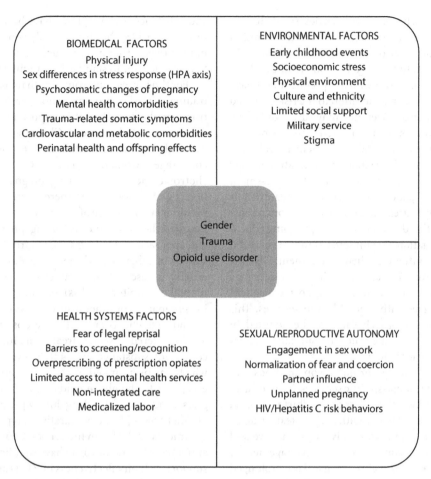

**Figure 5.2** Intersecting domains of current research: gender, trauma, and opioid-use disorder

trauma screening may prevent wasteful errors in diagnosis and treatment planning. For example, trauma self-report questionnaires can be administered in the relative privacy of a waiting room setting and may serve as an effective catalyst to the clinical interview. The number of items, completion times, and psychometric properties of many such screening tools are available to health professionals for comparative review [23, 24].

A trauma-informed lens may also be utilized when reviewing the general medical history. Frequent emergency department visits, injuries inconsistent with the stated history, missed appointments, late initiation of prenatal care, multiple unplanned pregnancies, or medication nonadherence may relate to gender-linked trauma. Additionally, among reproductive-aged women, a diagnosis of PTSD can also be significantly associated with chronic pain, gastrointestinal, and gynecologic problems [25]. Women with a history of

PTSD or PTSD and depression have also been found more likely to experience sexual dysfunction, genital pain, dyspareunia, menstrual abnormalities, and reproductive difficulties [26]. It may be important to discern if such trauma-related somatic symptoms may have historically been managed or masked with clinically prescribed opiates or benzodiazepines in addition to illicit drugs. PTSD has been found to correlate with prescription of opiates in pregnancy [27], and evidence suggests that benzodiazepines are now increasingly prescribed to women with PTSD as compared to their male peers [28].

As the gynecologic exam or childbirth itself may trigger feelings of fear or embarrassment among women with trauma histories and PTSD [29], preparatory discussion regarding exam procedures can elicit ways to reduce the patient's anticipated stress. A variety of potentially useful modification techniques in the context of a trauma history have been described [30, 31]. However some techniques, such as the administration of benzodiazepines prior to anticipated stressors in nonemergency settings, may be contraindicated for multiple reasons in those who are pregnant and have substance use disorder. In addition to the risks detailed in Chapter 4, benzodiazepines may also potentially precipitate or worsen trauma-related dissociation.

If the completed clinical assessment reveals that further mental health evaluation or treatment may be beneficial, the provider can review the assessment results with the patient. If referral to treatment is declined, it may be useful to explore the reasons or barriers related to this decision. However, ongoing education and reevaluation of symptoms at future visits can be offered and continued in lieu of treatment. Discreet referral to community-based or online resources may also provide alternative sources of support to a patient reluctant to engage with mental health services. This trauma-informed approach can also be adopted in circumstances where integrated or specialty mental health care is not accessible.

Regardless of whether or not a woman chooses to engage in direct trauma-specific services, it can be useful to understand whether labor or childbirth may also be perceived as a source of anticipatory fear or anxiety [32–35], and plan accordingly. A preemptive and collaborative discussion regarding the management of possible complications such as intense pain, prolonged labor, perineal tear, hemorrhage, and cesarean section can maximize a woman's sense of autonomy and control.

For pregnant women who desire mental health treatment but wish to avoid psychotropic medication, cognitive behavioral therapy can be therapeutic for this population [36], is likely safe in pregnancy [37, 38], and can be integrated successfully into primary care settings [39]. One form of cognitive behavioral therapy that seeks to address both trauma and substance use symptoms is Seeking Safety [40], which can be delivered in individual or in group formats. Seeking Safety may effectively reduce substance use symptoms in those women who are heavy substance users at baseline, and may also reduce HIV risk behaviors in substance-abusing women who engage more frequently in high-risk sexual activities at baseline [41]. Women whose PTSD symptoms respond to Seeking Safety may also be more likely to experience more global improvement in other mental health domains [42]. A number of other promising treatment programs for trauma-related

and substance use symptoms have been developed in recent years [43], but future study is needed to determine if these programs produce outcomes for women that are superior to standard community treatments.

For those pregnant women with moderate to severe trauma-related symptoms who wish to try psychotropic medication, first it is important to ask if there is future plan to breastfeed. Choosing an initial medication that minimizes infant drug exposure may help encourage a woman's adherence to a prescribed psychotropic medication during pregnancy and lactation. Furthermore, while there is little data to guide the clinician in the use of these medications in treating trauma-related symptoms during pregnancy, a general approach can be extrapolated from observational studies of other related mental health and sleep disorders, as described in Chapter 4. Selective serotonin reuptake inhibitors (SSRIs) are commonly used during pregnancy for other disorders, with comparatively few adverse effects and little overdose potential, and are considered first-line treatments for PTSD in the context of substance use [44]. However, paroxetine, which has been linked to congenital anomalies, is an exception to the above guidance and consensus suggests avoidance of this drug during pregnancy in favor of other SSRIs [45]. Comparatively, typical adjunctive treatments for PTSD in the general population such as antipsychotics and prazosin have significantly less data supporting their effectiveness in PTSD and their safety in pregnancy.

In summary, women experience significant vulnerability to trauma-related mental illnesses such as PTSD throughout the lifespan. For women of reproductive age, unique causal pathways of trauma can include aspects of pregnancy, labor, and childbirth. Additionally, women in this age group are concurrently entering into military roles and other traditionally male-dominated arenas where there is additional risk of trauma exposure. Potential opportunities for collaborative research include the need to better understand how women's experiences of trauma intersect with opioid-use disorder, and the need to improve treatment outcomes related not just to mental health, but also to physical and reproductive health.

# References

1. Grella C. E. From generic to gender-responsive treatment: changes in social policies, treatment services, and outcomes of women in substance abuse treatment. *J Psychoactive Drugs* 2008;40(Suppl 5):327–43.

2. American Psychiatric Association. *Diagnostic and Statistical Manual of Mental Disorders* (5th ed). Arlington, VA: American Psychiatric Publishing, 2013.

3. Kessler R. C., Sonnega A., Bromet E., Hughes M., Nelson C. B. Posttraumatic stress disorder in the National Comorbidity Survey. *Arch Gen Psychiatry* 1995;52(12):1048–60.

4. Pietrzak R. H., Goldstein R. B., Southwick S. M., Grant B. F. Prevalence and Axis I comorbidity of full and partial posttraumatic stress disorder in the United States: results from Wave 2 of the National Epidemiologic Survey on alcohol and related conditions. *J Anxiety Disord* 2011;25(3):456–65.

5. Mendez-Figueroa H., Dahlke J. D., Vrees R. A., Rouse D. J. Trauma in pregnancy: an updated systematic review. *Am J Obstet Gynecol* 2013 Jul;209(1):1–10.

6. Vesga-López O., Blanco C., Keyes K., et al. Psychiatric disorders in pregnant and postpartum women in the United States. *Arch Gen Psychiatry* 2008;65(7):805–15.

7. Seng J. S., Rauch S. A. M., Resnick H., et al. Exploring posttraumatic stress disorder symptom profile among pregnant women. *J Psychosom Obstet Gynecol* 2010 Sep;31(3):176–87.

8. Seng J. S., Low L. K., Sperlich M., Ronis D. L., Liberzon I. Post-traumatic stress disorder, child abuse history, birthweight and gestational age: a prospective cohort study. *BJOG* 2011 Oct;118(11):1329–39.

9. Yonkers K. A., Smith M. V., Forray A., et al. Pregnant women with posttraumatic stress disorder and risk of preterm birth. *JAMA Psychiatry* 2014;71(8):897–904.

10. Beck C. T., Gable R. K., Sakala C., Declercq E. R. Posttraumatic stress disorder in new mothers: results from a two-stage U.S. national survey. *Birth* 2011 Sep;38(3):216–27.

11. Yehuda R., Teicher M. H., Seckl J. R., et al. Parental posttraumatic stress disorder as a vulnerability factor for low cortisol trait in offspring of holocaust survivors. *Arch Gen Psychiatry* 2007 Sep;64(9):1040–8.

12. Torchalla I., Linden I. A., Strehlau V., Neilson E. K., Krausz M. "Like a lots happened with my whole childhood": violence, trauma, and addiction in pregnant and postpartum women from Vancouver's Downtown Eastside. *Harm Reduct J* 2015;(12):1.

13. Smith K. Z., Smith P. H., Cercone S. A., McKee S. A., Homish G. G. Past year non-medical opioid use and abuse and PTSD diagnosis: interactions with sex and associations with symptom clusters. *Addict Behav* 2016 Jul;58:167–74.

14. Peirce J. M., Schacht R. L., Brooner R. K., King V. L., Kidorf M. S. Prospective risk factors for traumatic event reexposure in community syringe exchange participants. *Drug Alcohol Depend* 2014 May 1;138:98–102.

15. Erickson S., Tonigan J. Trauma and intravenous drug use among pregnant alcohol/other drug abusing women: factors in predicting child abuse potential. *Alcsm Treat Quart* 2008;26(3):313–32.

16. Rinehart D. J., Becker M. A., Buckley P. R., et al. The relationship between mothers' child abuse potential and current mental health symptoms: implications for screening and referral. *J Behav Health Serv Res* 2005 Apr–Jun;32(2):155–66.

17. Greaves L., Poole N., Boyle E. *Transforming Addiction: Gender, Trauma, Transdisciplinarity*. New York, NY and East Sussex: Routledge, 2015.

18. Terplan M., Longinaker N., Appel L. Women-centered drug treatment services and need in the United States, 2002–2009. *Am J Public Health* 2015 Nov;105(11):e50–4.

19. Substance Abuse and Mental Health Services Administration. Trauma-Informed Care in Behavioral Health Services. *Treatment Improvement Protocol (TIP) Series 57. HHS Publication No. (SMA) 13-4801.* Rockville, MD: Substance Abuse and Mental Health Services Administration, 2014, Appendices B and F: 247–65, 287.

20. Loveland Cook C. A., Flick L. H., Homan S. M., et al. Posttraumatic stress disorder in pregnancy: prevalence, risk factors, and treatment. *Obstet Gynecol* 2004 Apr;103(4):710–7.

21. Smith M. V., Poschman K., Kessler Cavaleri M. A., Howell H. B., Yonkers K. A. Symptoms of posttraumatic stress disorder in a community sample of low-income pregnant women. *Am J Psychiatry* 2006;163:881–4.

22. Killeen T. K., Back S. E., Brady K. T. Implementation of integrated therapies for comorbid post-traumatic stress disorder and substance use disorders in community substance abuse treatment programs. *Drug Alcohol Rev* 2015;34:234–41.

23. Substance Abuse and Mental Health Services Administration. Trauma-Informed Care in Behavioral Health Services. *Treatment Improvement Protocol (TIP) Series 57. HHS Publication No. (SMA) 13-4801.* Rockville, MD: Substance Abuse and Mental Health Services Administration, 2014, Appendix D: 271–84.

24. PTSD: National Center for PTSD Home. For Professionals: Assessment Overview. Available at: www.ptsd.va.gov/professional/assessment/overview/index.asp. Retrieved January 14, 2017.

25. Seng J. S., Clark M. K., McCarthy A. M., Ronis D. L. PTSD and physical comorbidity among women receiving Medicaid: results from service-use data. *J Trauma Stress* 2006 Feb;19(1):45–56.

26. Cohen B. E., Maguen S., Bertenthal D., Shi Y., Jacoby V., Seal K. H. Reproductive and other health outcomes in Iraq and Afghanistan women veterans using VA health care: association with

mental health diagnoses. *Womens Health Issues* 2012 Sep;22(5):e461–71.

27. Smith M. V., Costello D., Yonkers K. A. Clinical correlates of prescription opioid analgesic use in pregnancy. *Matern Child Health J* 2015 Mar;19(3):548–56.

28. Bernardy N. C., Lund B. C., Alexander B., Jenkyn A. B., Schnurr P. P., Friedman M. J. (2013). Gender differences in prescribing among veterans diagnosed with posttraumatic stress disorder. *J Gen Intern Med* 28(Suppl 2):542–8.

29. Weitlauf J. C., Finney J. W., Ruzek J. I., et al. Distress and pain during pelvic examinations: effect of sexual violence. *Obstet Gynecol* 2008 Dec;112(6):1343–50.

30. Bates C. K., Carroll N., Potter J. The challenging pelvic examination. *J Gen Intern Med* 2011 Jun;26(6):651–7.

31. Adult manifestations of childhood sexual abuse. ACOG (American College of Obstetricians and Gynecologists) committee opinion, number 498, August 2011.

32. Modarres M., Afrasiabi S., Rahnama P., Montazeri A. Prevalence and risk factors of childbirth-related post-traumatic stress symptoms. *BMC Pregnancy Childbirth* 2012;12:88.

33. Grekin R., O'Hara M. W. Prevalence and risk factors of postpartum posttraumatic stress disorder: a meta-analysis. *Clin Psychol Rev* 2014 Jul;34(5):389–401.

34. Ayers S. Thoughts and emotions during traumatic birth: a qualitative study. *Birth* 2007;34:253–63.

35. Harris R., Ayers S. What makes labour and birth traumatic? A survey of intrapartum 'hotspots'. *Psychol Health* 2012;27(10):1166–77.

36. Cohen L.R., Hien D.A. Treatment outcomes for women with substance abuse and PTSD who have experienced complex trauma. *Psychiatr Serv (Washington, DC)* 2006;57(1):100–6.

37. Lilliecreutz C., Josefsson A., Sydsjo G. An open trial with cognitive behavioral therapy for blood – and

injection phobia in pregnant women – a group intervention program. *Arch Womens Ment Health* 2010 Jun;13(3):259–65.

38. Arch J. J., Dimidjian S., Chessick C. Are exposure-based cognitive behavioral therapies safe during pregnancy? *Arch Womens Ment Health* 2012 Dec;15(6):445–7.

39. Roy-Byrne P., Craske M. G., Sullivan G., et al. Delivery of evidence-based treatment for multiple anxiety disorders in primary care: a randomized controlled trial. *JAMA: J Am Med Assoc.* 2010 May;303(19):1921–8.

40. Najavits L. M. *Seeking Safety: A Treatment Manual for PTSD and Substance Abuse.* New York: Guilford Press, 2002.

41. Hien D. A., Campbell A. N. C., Killeen T. et al. The impact of trauma-focused group therapy upon HIV sexual risk behaviors in the NIDA Clinical Trials Network "Women and Trauma" Multi-Site Study. *AIDS Behav* 2010 Apr;14(2):421–30.

42. Hien D. A., Jiang H., Campbell A. N. C., et al. Do treatment improvements in PTSD severity affect substance use outcomes? A secondary analysis from a randomized clinical trial in NIDA's Clinical Trials Network. *Am J Psychiatr* 2010 Jan;167(1):95–101.

43. Substance Abuse and Mental Health Services Administration. Trauma-Informed Care in Behavioral Health Services. *Treatment Improvement Protocol (TIP) Series 57. HHS Publication No. (SMA) 13-4801.* Rockville, MD: Substance Abuse and Mental Health Services Administration, 2014, 137–55.

44. Shorter D., Hsieh J., Kosten T. R. Pharmacologic management of comorbid post-traumatic stress disorder and addictions. *Am J Addict* 2015 Dec;24(8):705–12.

45. ACOG Committee on Practice Bulletins – Obstetrics. Use of psychiatric medications during pregnancy and lactation. *Obstet Gynecol* 2008 Apr;111(4):1001–20.

# Intimate Partner Violence, Pregnancy and Substance Use Disorder

Richard G. Soper and Hendrée E. Jones

## Introduction and Defining Intimate Partner Violence

The issues of substance use disorder, interpersonal violence and pregnancy are often intertwined and cannot be treated in isolation. Intimate partner violence (IPV), also called domestic violence (DV), is defined as: Behavior that results in emotional, physical, sexual, or psychological harm to a current or former partner or spouse (including common-law spouse), dating partner, or boy/girlfriend. IPV occurs in all races, ethnicities, sexual identity and orientation, and social and economic levels of society. IPV is neither a spontaneous act of anger nor a one-time occurrence [1, 2]. Intimate partner violence impacts an estimated one in four women, and one in eight men across the lifespan, resulting in numerous mental, physical, and reproductive health consequences (Figure 6.1).

Substance use disorder has been found to co-occur in 40–60 percent of IPV incidents across various studies. A review of the characteristics of 2,729 women enrolled in treatment programs designed to integrate trauma-informed services with services for co-occurring substance use and mental health disorders found that approximately 75 percent of these women experienced multiple and repeated abuses, including sexual abuse, physical abuse, and emotional abuse and neglect. The average age of initial sexual and physical abuse was 13 years of age, while the age of onset for emotional and physical neglect was nine years of age [3]. Such a pervasive history of trauma has significant implications for health service delivery practices on several levels. Pregnant women with substance use disorder are more likely to be in a current or recent intimate partner violence (IPV) relationship than pregnant women without such a disorder [4]. An interwoven and strong relationship between substance use disorder and perpetration of IPV has been found in numerous primary care healthcare settings, including prenatal clinics, family practice settings, rural and urban healthcare clinics,

substance use disorder treatment centers and psychiatric settings [2]. The ripple effects of IPV extend well beyond health care, affecting interpersonal, familial, community, educational, occupational, and societal functioning. IPV strains all the legal, medical, cultural and societal resources [5, 6]. This chapter first reviews the inter-relationship between IPV, substance use disorder and pregnancy. Next discussed is the context that keeps victims and perpetrators of violence within the abusive relationship followed by a summary of ways to identify, assess and respond to a woman with IPV, substance use disorder, and pregnancy.

## Who is At Risk for IPV?

Primary health care professionals may overlook IPV due to a number of factors including, age, lack of awareness, misconceptions, lack of education, time constraints, risk liability, as well as other factors. Rarely are senior age patients, male or female, evaluated for IPV. IPV is a risk for all age populations [6]. It is important to know the risk factors for IPV so that those who are suffering can be identified and helped. Below are some known risk factors for IPV:

- Verbal abuse is the single variable most likely to predict IPV [1].
- Prior history of IPV victimization is often seen in perpetrators.
- Racial and ethnic minorities experience higher rates of IPV than whites [7].
- The rates of IPV do not significantly differ in urban or rural locations.
- Same gender relationships may also be at higher risk for IPV than opposite gender relationships. In same gender relationships, frequently an inaccurate assumption is that there is equal control or strength in the partners and/or when there is evidence of violence, it was not deliberate. However, data for rates amongst lesbian, gay, bisexual, transgender (LGBT) persons are difficult

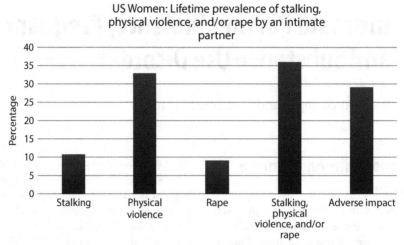

US Women: Lifetime prevalence of stalking, physical violence, and/or rape by an intimate partner

Adverse impact would include: injury, health care provider or counseling contact, fear, safety concerns, PTSD symptoms, loss of work; for those women who reported being raped it also includes having contracted a sexually transmitted disease or having become pregnant.

**Figure 6.1** Lifetime prevalence of IPV of Women in the United States
*Source*: National Intimate Partner and Sexual Violence Survey, 2010

to assess with very limited reporting and study biases to date [2, 5].

- Women compared to men, regardless of sexual orientation, have a higher incidence of IPV. Intimate partners can be of same or opposite gender [8].
- Spousal abuse has been identified as a predictor of developing a substance use disorder [1, 2].
- One of the strongest correlated risk factors for future aggression by both males and females is a history of previous partner aggression [9].
- In some relationships, the issue of mutual aggression may also be occurring.

In a study of pregnant patients in North Carolina, victims of IPV were significantly more likely to use multiple substances before and during pregnancy than those who had no experience of IPV. This study also found that on days of heavy drug and/or alcohol use, physical violence was 11 times more likely among IPV batterers and victims [10].

## The Interconnection between IPV and Other Life Stressors

Distinct connections between IPV and several issues cannot be overlooked. Figure 6.2 shows examples of the co-occurring issues that are associated with IPV.

- Depression
- Substance use disorder
- Homelessness
- Poverty
- Stress
- Unemployment
- Past childhood history of physical, sexual and/or emotional abuse
- Past adult history of physical, sexual and/or emotional abuse

**Figure 6.2** Co-occurring issues linked to IPV

Of note, past history of childhood sexual abuse (CSA) increases the likelihood of sexual victimization as an adult [8, 11]. That said, many people who experience such situations never become perpetrators or victims of IPV. Similarly, resolution of these issues may not stop or reduce IPV [12–14].

People experiencing and surviving IPV often turn to alcohol, drugs or other substances/behaviors to cope with abuse; substance use disorders/addiction can, in turn, decrease inhibitions and increase risk of further violence. IPV affects the whole family unit; children in the home where IPV occurs and extended family suffer serious adverse effects in childhood and adulthood, creating additional burden on the healthcare system [15]. Verbal and physical abuse has profound effects on self-esteem and can affect mental and physical health outcomes as a result.

## The Morbidity and Lethality of IPV

Every healthcare professional must take seriously the great harm that IPV inflicts on those individuals experiencing it. Clinical outcomes in those individuals experiencing IPV are wide ranging and can include, but are not limited to, fractures, head trauma, chronic gynecological conditions, somatic disorders, co-occurring neurological and/or psychiatric disorders (e.g., PTSD), and suicide. Further, IPV can have a negative impact on the immune system [8], and may negatively affect medication adherence and lead to exacerbation of disease effects including those of substance use disorder. Further, the below bullets highlight critical harms of IPV.

- Survivors of IPV are twice as likely to attempt suicide multiple times and causes of murder/suicide are most likely to occur in the context of IPV [11, 16].
- Over 50 percent of intimate partner violence survivors are strangled at some point in the course of the relationship – often repeatedly, over years and the overwhelming majority of strangulation perpetrators are men.
- The victims strangled to the point of losing consciousness are at high risk of dying within the first 24–48 hours after the incident from cerebral vascular accident, aspiration, blunt force trauma and/or thromboembolism. Such incidents cause traumatic brain injury (TBI).
- The vast majority of IPV victims showing signs of TBI never receive a formal diagnosis [11]. The act of strangulation is the penultimate abuse by a perpetrator prior to a homicide. Yet, today only 38 states prosecute strangulation as a felony. For many survivors, IPV leads to post traumatic stress disorder (PTSD) [17, 18].

The interwoven and connected effects of these conditions have significant impact on health care. These syndemics, the presence of two diseases that interact and exacerbate the negative health effects of one or both of the diseases, are the consequential interactions of substance abuse/addiction, trauma including violence and other conditions [19, 20].

## The Context Bonding Perpetrators and Victims of Violence within the Abusive Relationship: Trauma Bonded

People in violent relationships frequently remain in the relationship for numerous reasons. Figure 6.3 lists

- Love for the perpetrator, even after a violent event
- Lack of financial support
- Isolation
- Stigma, shame and prejudice from family, community, religion
- Language barriers
- Coercer for dependent minors
- Fear of consequences for the perpetrator
- Fear of self or children being taken, harmed
- The concept of "trauma-bonding"
- Pregnancy

**Figure 6.3** Examples of reasons keeping the victim with the perpetrator

examples of the diverse array of reasons why victims stay with perpetrators. Bonding is a biological and emotional process that makes people more important to each other over time. Bonding is not something that can be lost, unlike love, trust, attraction. Bonding is cumulative. Experiencing, together, extreme situations and extreme feelings tends to bond people in a unique way. Trauma bonding is the misuse of fear, excitement, sexual feelings, and sexual physiology to entangle another person [21–23]. Trauma bonding occurs when the target (victim) feels emotionally and physically dependent on the abusive person (perpetrator) who rewards the target to make them believe the perpetrator is all-powerful. Trauma bonding is used to gain control over the victim (target) and can include control over all aspects of life. Alcohol and drug misuse can complicate motivation to leave an abusive or violent partner, if he/she is providing the drug or alcohol or sharing with the victim. Compounding these challenges is the fear that leaving will not make the survivor any safer. Termination of a relationship can explode into violence [7, 13].

Pregnancy is also a very significant complicating factor in IPV; an unwanted pregnancy can lead to escalation of the violence and abuse. An unexpected pregnancy can also lead to forced starvation, eating disorders, physical impairments, self-harm (cutting), alcohol and/or substance use disorder, and other chronic medical issues. Miscarriages and abortions can be forced and/or induced by the perpetrator. Perpetrators may restrict and/or monitor all aspects of a victim's life. Abusers frequently also control the financial resources, transportation, nutrition, clothing, bathing, sleeping, activities inside or outside the domicile, as well as access to medical care, severely limiting the victim's ability or willingness to leave. The strongest predictor of whether a victim will permanently separate or stay in the relationship is what, if any, access to adequate financial resources are available to the victim, independent of the perpetrator [17].

# Screening and Assessing for IPV Risk

Evidence suggests that if IPV is identified, brief clinical interventions focused on providing universal education about healthy relationships, routine inquiry about violence exposure, and brief counseling may be promising strategies for increasing awareness about violence, reducing isolation survivors feel, and, in some populations, reducing violence victimization. Addressing IPV is complicated because of social, ethnic, cultural, and religious stigma. No one wants to discuss this issue. Yet, understanding IPV and the syndemics that accompany it has significant implications for effective risk reduction and improving health outcomes, especially in women of childbearing age. The task of screening, treating or referring of IPV survivors can seem staggering. Healthcare professionals and law enforcement professionals who are trained in this issue are then better able to assist with this public health issue. The US Preventative Services Task Force (USPSTF) issued a recommendation in 2013 for primary care clinicians to screen women of childbearing age for IPV and refer any patient to intervention services that has a positive screen [24]. The statement only mentions women of childbearing age. It is imperative to remember women of any age and in any relationship can be at risk. Screening and assessing history of IPV, childhood sexual abuse and PTSD offers an opportunity to implement interventions early and has the potential to improve outcomes. There is no evidence that screening has caused harm to a patient.

The axiom, "FIRST DO NO HARM" should be followed, as always, when screening. Several guidelines are suggested. The following list is suggested as components that IPV screening program should have:[24]

- Written protocol and screening policies
- Documentation (progress notes, chart) using body maps or photos of injuries
- Protocols for reporting and referrals (if made)
- Staff training and local community education
- In-house IPV counselors/advocates
- Availability of prevention/intervention information

- Coordination among IPV, mental health and substance abuse providers with available support groups and services
- Linkage with community resources

No matter how healthcare professionals execute a program for screening and support, the goal should always be the same: keep the patient safe, healthy and do no harm.

The following list provides how to screen patients for IPV:

- Never screen in the presence of a possible perpetrator. Should the partner be in the room, request they leave, and defer screening until they have left. Request another member of staff escort the partner to another room or the waiting area. Always maintain safety for the patient. If an interpreter is necessary, language and sign services should be provided by someone unknown to the patient [17].
- It is mandatory to maintain respectful, empathic, nonjudgmental statements and questions with the patient. Provide emotional support. Know community resources and referrals.
- Screen in pairs. Always have another staff member in the room with the patient during the screening (optimally not same gender as perpetrator).
- Integrate screening questions into routine intake questions, possibly in social or family section, to diminish the stress/fear of the patient (i.e., due to violence being so prevalent these days, I ask all patients if they have been hurt by someone close to them).
- Keep the questions nonjudgmental and simple (i.e., Do you feel safe at home? How do you and your companion handle disagreements?).
- If part of the practice includes pediatric patients, consider using some screening questions during well-child or any trauma examination. (i.e., How are things at home?).
- How you ask matters. If the patient is reluctant to respond verbally, consider integrating a format where they can respond in writing (in intake form) or on the computer.
- Physical signs of trauma are sentinel events and the examination should incorporate questions about violence (i.e., How did this happen? Was anyone else involved?). If there is hesitancy, stay respectful of boundaries and cease the questioning. Return to the questions at a later point in the exam. Also leave open to the patient

an offer to explain in writing or discussion. Remember to always include a comprehensive physical exam including cranium when violence is suspected [25, 26].

- Know when and how to refer in your practice community and regional support resources for violence, including hotlines, mental health centers, safe houses/shelters, trained therapists, and develop a method to transfer a patient "safely" in those cases where you assess high risk of continuation of violence.

- Provide resources in lobby, patient exam, and waiting areas during patient appointments. Such resources should include telephone numbers and/or addresses for local food banks, suicide and violence hotlines (see Resources), law enforcement, shelters and others. Consider providing numbers in a discrete, small printout that patient can keep concealed.

- If the patient is able to discuss the situation with you, explore resource options with the patient. Remember financial resources are the number one reason victims stay in a violent situation.

- Know your state laws regarding mandatory reporting and become familiar with the Violence Against Women Act [27, 28]. Currently many states still define domestic violence (IPV) as a male-perpetrated violence against females. A 2002 study by the US Department of Justice found that most victims injured by an intimate partner did not seek professional medical treatment or report the injuries [29]. Many states still do not acknowledge Lesbian, Gay, Bisexual, Transgender (LGBT) relationships, lacking a system to deal with violence involving LGBT persons. As a consequence, in such states, IPV in several segments of the population is not reported due to such limitations, stigma, and discrimination. Statutes still exist, in many states, requiring a male/female relationship of offender/victim for filing a protective order [2]. A widespread lack of education and training amongst legal, medical, clergy, social services, entertainment (sports, etc.) and educational systems regarding IPV continues to exist worldwide, including in the United States [9, 30].

- Use screening tools – There are several studies that demonstrate patients will disclose IPV on a computer screen or on paper more freely than in conversation. The USPSTF has validated six brief tools that can be used to screen patients [24–26]. Consider adding one of the tools to the patient health questionnaire (PHQ) used to screen for depression.

- There is an IPV screening tool to use in the emergency room that aims to identify victims of IPV with a potential for traumatic brain injury (TBI), named HELPPS, although it has not been standardized as a tool, as of this date.

- A standard protocol for IPV screening questions, gender neutral is optimal. Guidelines can also be found at: www.accesscontinuingeducation.com/ACE4000/c7/index.htm.

- Integrate standardized screening methods to assess PTSD and other stress and anxiety disorders, such as Beck Depression Inventory, Post-traumatic Stress Checklist and the Stanford Acute Stress Questionnaire.

IPV screenings in a safe and accepting environment can increase a patient's willingness to discuss personal or medical information. The clinical value of screening for IPV has been endorsed by the American Medical Association and other major professional organizations. The American Association of Colleges of Nursing has published guidelines [31].

## Treating IPV among Women with Substance Use Disorders during Pregnancy

Health systems throughout the country have come to recognize that to address the needs of this vulnerable population, the service delivery system must integrate knowledge about IPV and substance use into systems of care, better known as trauma-informed services. These efforts are reflected in and supported by the National Center for Trauma Informed Care, a technical assistance center within the Substance Abuse Mental Health Services Administration, DHHS (2012).

To be "trauma-informed" means

1. Understanding the role that violence and victimization play in the lives of women seeking substance use and mental health services;

2. Designing a service system to accommodate the vulnerabilities of trauma survivors;

3. Delivering services in a manner that will facilitate participation in treatment [32]. This definition touches on several of the elements that need to be included in a trauma-informed system of care.

Programs should include a trauma policy or position statement within their policies and procedures to formalize their commitment to providing trauma-informed services. The policies and services must reflect a respect for culture, race, ethnicity, gender, age, sexual orientation, and physical disability. There should be specific trauma-related practice guidelines and treatment approaches, including procedures to avoid re-traumatization. Program staff, including non-clinical staff, need to have specialized training related to trauma so that they are sensitive to the vulnerabilities of trauma survivors, with trauma-informed competencies included in their job standards. Programs need to ensure that the experiences and perspectives of trauma survivors are represented in the development and implementation of services, and specialized trauma programs need to be integrated within mental health and substance use services [33].

Steps a provider can take to assist women in seeking safety from IPV:

- Acknowledging the abuse. Directly and clearly state that the abuse has happened and/or continues to happen and such abuse is against her human rights.
- Safety plan. Determine the woman's desire to develop a plan. Ask her to identify people she trusts who live very close to her home (e.g., neighbors) or others (e.g., family, friends) and develop a code with them that she can use to alert them when she is in danger and they should call for help. If the plan includes leaving, help her determine steps to take for her safety and the safety of her children. How will she access money? Transportation? Clothing? Personal identification and personal documents?
- Any materials that the provider gives the patient should be disguised. For example, phone numbers for services should be embedded in other material that abusers are not interested in or that look innocuous.
- Containment. Plans should be made and strategies should be suggested to the patient for how she can protect herself from further abuse or from an escalation of the abuse.
- Support/Affirm. Acknowledge the abuse and emphasize that no one deserves to be treated this way. Affirm that there is hope for the future and that she is not alone in this experience or in leaving this potentially life-threatening situation.

- Focus on coping. Some providers fear that by discussing the problem they will re-traumatize the patient. To lower this risk, rather than asking for details about the abuse or violence exposure, the provider needs to focus on the present situation and the skills the patient can be taught to cope, what has happened and what she can do to avoid future abuse.
- Referral. Clinics should have an updated list of referrals to community or national violence exposure services to give to patients. As noted above, any materials given to the patient must be disguised so they do not raise the suspicion of the abuser and risk bringing greater harm to the patient.

Trauma-specific services differ from trauma-informed services in that they are designed to treat the actual sequelae of abuse trauma. There are several trauma-specific service models that have been validated through research and are considered best-practice models. The following are models that are widely used in treatment programs for women:

- Seeking Safety: A Treatment Manual for PTSD and Substance Abuse ([34]; www.seekingsafety.org).
- Trauma Recovery and Empowerment Model (TREM; [35]; www.ccdc1.org).
- Beyond Trauma: A Healing Journey for Women ([36]; www.stephaniecovington.com).
- The Sanctuary Model ([37]; www.sanctuaryweb.com).

## Summary

Substance use disorder, interpersonal violence (IPV) and pregnancy are commonly intertwined issues. Pregnancy is not a protective factor from IPV; in some cases, it can increase IPV. Intimate partner violence is the leading cause of female homicides and injury-related deaths during pregnancy and accounts for significant preventable injuries and emergency department visits by women. IPV is among the most frequently fatal and under-treated issue today. The ripple effects of IPV extend well beyond health care, affecting interpersonal, familial, community, educational, occupational, and societal functioning. IPV strains all the legal, medical, cultural and societal resources. There are known risk factors that healthcare providers must screen for and then respond to when the screen is positive. The benefits of screening and interventions go well beyond the patient. IPV affects the whole family unit. The Kaiser ACE project/study of adverse childhood experiences has well-documented the impact of IPV on childhood and the lifelong sequelae [24]. Kaiser Permanente North California (KPNC) has, for over 15 years, made inquiry, recognition and intervention of IPV "part of everyday care." One component of the KPNC system is visible messaging for patients throughout the health center (Posters: "Are You being hurt? We can help, talk to your doctor) [38, 39]. The long-term sustainability of intimate violence (IPV) prevention requires clear alignment with other health care priorities, such as patient safety, care coordination, efficiency, and improved patient outcomes. This helps to ensure that health care decision makers see this as an area of positive investment as stated by Kaiser Permanente Medical Group CEO "Intimate partner violence prevention is a part of a strategic approach to quality service and affordability. By doing the right thing, we can improve quality outcomes, patient satisfaction, and the personal lives of our patients while decreasing the cost to employers and individuals" [39].

# References

1. American Psychological Association. *Intimate partner violence: facts and resources.* Available at: www.apa.org/topics/violence/partner.aspx. Retrieved September 16, 2016.

2. O'Doherty L. J., Taft A., Hagarty K., et al. Screening women for intimate partner violence in healthcare settings: abridged Cochran systematic review and meta-analysis. *BMJ* 2014;348:q2913.

3. Becker M. A., Noether C. D., Larson M. J., et al. Characteristics of women engaged in treatment for trauma and co-occurring disorders: findings from a national multi-site study. *J Community Psychol* 2005;33(4):429–43.

4. Engstrom M., El-Bassel N., Gilbert L. Childhood sexual abuse characteristics, intimate partner violence exposure and psychological distress among women in methadone treatment. *J Subst Abuse Treat* 2012;43(3):366–76.

5. Lunine B. American Bar Association Commission on Domestic Violence. Transitioning your services: serving transgender victims of domestic violence, sexual assault and stalking. *e-Newsletter* 2008:11(Summer). Available at: www.abanet.org/domviol/enewsletter/vol11/expert2.html. Retrieved February 19, 2015.

6. Catalano S. M. Intimate partner violence in the United States, Intimate Partner Violence 1993–2010 (September 29, 2015). NCJ 239203. Available at: www.bjs.gov/content/pub/pdf/ipv9310.pdf. Retrieved November 11, 2016.

7. Tjaden P., Thoennes N. U.S. Department of Justice. Extent, nature, and consequences of intimate partner violence: research project. 2000. Available at: www.ncjrs.gov/pdffiles1/nij/181867.pdf. Retrieved August 7, 2016.

8. Centers for Disease Control and Prevention (CDC). Definition of intimate partner violence. October 21, 2008. Available at: www.cdc.gov/ViolencePrevention?intimatepartnerviolence/definitions.html. Retrieved August 7, 2016.

9. Adler N. E., Johnson P. A. Violence and women's health. *Science* 2015;350(6258):257.

10. Martin S. L., English K. T., Clark K. A., Cilenti D., Kupper L. L. Violence and substance use among North Carolina pregnant women. *Am J Pub Health* 1996;887:991–8.

11. Zink T., Regan S., Goldenhar L., et al. Intimate partner violence: what are physicians perspectives? *J Am Board of Fam Practice* 2004;17(5):332–40.

12. Zierler S. University of California, San Francisco AIDS Health Project. Violence and HIV: strategies for primary and secondary prevention. *Focus* 2001;16(6):1–4.

13. Pajouhi P. University of California, San Francisco AIDS Project. Domestic violence. *HIV Counselor Perspective* 2000;9(4):1–8.

14. Centers for Disease Control and Prevention (CDC). Understanding intimate partner violence (fact sheet). 2006. Available at: www.cdc.gov/ncipc/dvp/ipv_factsheet.pdf. Retrieved August 7, 2016.

15. Felitti V. J., Anda R. F., Nordenberg D., et al. Relationship of childhood abuse and household dysfunction to many of the leading causes of death in adults. *Am J Prev Med* 1998;14(4):248–58. Available at: www.ajponline.org/article/s0749-3797(98)00017-8/abstract. Retrieved November 11, 2016.

16. Soper R. Intimate partner violence and co-occurring substance abuse/addiction. *Paradigm* 2016;20(4):20–1. Available at: www.addictionrecov.org/Paradigm/DisplayParadigmIssue.aspx? Retrieved December 10, 2016.

17. Myers H. F., Wyatt G. E., Loeb T. B., et al. Severity of child sexual abuse, post-traumatic stress and risky sexual behavior among HIV positive women. *AIDS Behavior* 2006;10(2):191–9.

18. New York State Department of Health. *Guidelines for integrating domestic violence screening into counseling, testing, referral and partner notification.* 2002. Available at: www.health.state.ny.us/nysdoh/rfa/hiv/guide.htm. Retrieved February 12, 2015.

19. Center for Disease Control and Prevention (CDC). *Syndemics overview history: what is syndemic?* 2008. Available at: www.cdc.gov/syndemics/overview-history.htm. Retrieved February 17, 2015.

20. Scott-Storey K. Cumulative abuse: do all things add up? *Trauma, Violence Abuse* 2011;12(3);135–50.

21. Trauma Bonded-definition. Available at: www.abuseandrelationships.org/Content/Survivors/trauma_bonding.html. Retrieved October 30, 2016.

22. Carnes P. *Don't call it love.* New York, NY: Penguin Random House; 1992.

23. Carnes P. *Trauma bonds.* Available at: www.themeadows.com/workshops/the-betrayal-bond-breaking-free of-exploitive-relationships. Retrieved November 11, 2016.

24. Meyer V. A. US Preventative Services Task Force. Screening for intimate partner violence and abuse of elderly and vulnerable adults: US Preventative Task Force recommendation statement. *Ann Intern Med* 2013:(158);478–86.

25. U.S. Government Printing Office. 113th congress of the United States of America. Violence against women reauthorization act of 2013. Available at: www.gpo.gov/fdsys/pkg/FR-2014-10-20/pdf/2014-24284.pdf. Fact Sheet; Available at: www.whitehouse.gov/sites/default/files/docs/vawa_factsheet.pdf. Retrieved November 11, 2016.

26. American Academy of Orthopaedic Surgeons/American Association of Orthopaedic Surgeons. *Family violence state statutes.* Available at: http://aaos.org/about/abuse/ststatut.asp. Retrieved November 11, 2016.

27. Miller E., McCaw B., Humphreys B. L., Mitchell C. Integrating intimate partner violence assessment and intervention into health care in the United States: a systems approach. *J Women's Health* (Larchmt) 2015;24(1):92–9.

28. McCow B. *Using a systems model approach to improving intimate partner violence services in a large healthcare organization. Preventing violence against women and children workshop summary.* Washington, DC: National Academics Press; 2011. p. 169–84.

29. US Department of Justice, Office of Justice Programs, National Institute of Justice. *Documenting domestic violence: how health care providers can help victims.* Available at: www.ncjrs.gov/pdffiles1/nij/188564.pdf. Retrieved November 11, 2016.

30. Chermack S. T., Murray R. L., Winters J. J., Walton M. A., Booth B. M., Blow F. C. Treatment needs of men and women with violence problems in substance use disorder treatment. *Subst Use Misuse* 2009;(44):1236–62.

31. Black M. C., Basile K. C., Breitling M. J., et al. *The national intimate partner and sexual violence survey 2010 summary report.* Atlantic: National Center for Injury Prevention and Control, Center for Disease Control and Prevention; 2011. Available at: www.cdc.gov/violenceprevention/pdf/nisvs_report2010-a.pdf. Retrieved October 30, 2016.

32. Harris M., Fallot R. (Eds.) *New directions for mental health services: Using trauma theory to design service systems, No. 89.* San Francisco, CA: Jossey Bass; 2001.

33. Blanch A. *Developing trauma-informed behavioral systems: Report from NTAC's national experts meeting on Trauma and Violence.* Alexandria, VA: US Department of Health and Human Services, Substance Abuse and Mental Health Services Administration; 2003.

34. Najavits L. M. *Seeking safety: a treatment manual for PTSD and substance abuse.* New York, NY: Guilford; 2002.

35. Fallot R. D., Harris M. The Trauma Recovery Empowerment Model (TREM): conceptual and practical issues in a group intervention for women. *Community Ment Health* 38(6):475–85.

36. Covington S. *Beyond trauma: a healing journey for women.* Center City, MN: Hazelden; 2003.

37. Bloom S. The sanctuary model: developing generic inpatient programs for the treatment of psychological trauma. In Williams MB, Sommer JF. (Eds.), *Handbook of post-traumatic therapy: a practical guide to intervention, treatment, and research.* Westport, CT: Greenwood Pub.; 1994. p. 474–91.

38. Nankin J., Dietzen L., Sangsland S., Eshilian-Oates L. At the nexus of substance use disorder and intimate partner violence. *Advances in Addiction & Recovery* 2014;Fall:18–23.

39. Pence B. W., Reif S., Whetten K., et al. Minorities, the poor, and survivors of abuse: HIV-infected patients in the US deep south. *South Med J* 2007;100(11):1114–22.

## Hotlines

National Domestic Violence Hotline: 800-799-SAFE (7233)

Rape Abuse & Incest National Network (RAINN): 800-656-HOPE (4673)

## Websites (Retrieved January 6, 2017)

Futures without Violence www.futureswithoutviolence.org

Violence Education Tools Online (VETO violence) www.cdc.gov/violenceprevention/fundedprograms/veto.html

Mary Kay Foundation www.marykayfoundation.org

National Coalition Against Domestic Violence www.ncadv.org

National Network to End Domestic Violence www.nnedv.org

Office on Violence Against Women (US Department of Justice) www.justice.gov/ovw

# Medical Comorbidities in Women with Opioid Use Disorders in Pregnancy

Kaylin A. Klie

## Introduction

Providing medical care, prenatal or otherwise, to a pregnant woman with substance use disorder is a unique opportunity to address immediate medical concerns, and also to attend to health issues that may have gone unnoticed or ignored during active use. Many people, and particularly pregnant women, with substance use disorder are hesitant to seek routine medical care. In fact, assessments of utilization of health care repeatedly demonstrate that people with substance misuse, "heavy" alcohol use, and/or intravenous substance use receive less preventative and routine health care for minor ailments than any other demographic [1], despite having similar rates of need of treatment for chronic medical and mental health conditions as nonsubstance using people [2].

## General Medical History

Beginning with the initial prenatal visit, taking a thorough medical history should include all the categories of assessment regularly employed for all patients, including current concerns, allergies, medications, review of systems, past medical history, past surgical history, family and social history [3]. The first interview should, naturally, also include a thorough obstetrical and gynecological history. Given the time and attention, this type of history gathering can make this as an excellent opportunity for rapport building prior to more in-depth questions regarding substance use.

## Substance Use History

In addition to these usual assessments, a thorough substance use history should be obtained with compassion and acceptance, paying special attention to history of withdrawal symptoms and/or prior hospitalizations or treatments needed for detoxification complications. As described in earlier chapters, many pregnant women have a history of polysubstance use, and careful attention should be employed to assess for need for level of care if detoxification is necessary. For example, women with use of opioids as well as benzodiazepines and/or alcohol may have history of complicated withdrawal. Knowing this information will help the prenatal provider assess for necessary referral for residential or inpatient detoxification.

## Physical Exam

Keeping in mind the significant number of women with history of emotional, physical, and/or sexual trauma who develop substance use disorders, providing a comprehensive prenatal physical exam should be completed with the patient's safety and comfort in mind. This should include a discussion of what body parts need to be examined prior to physically contacting the patient, providing the option of patient moving or adjusting clothing, or undressing in stages, instead of completely undressing and wearing a gown, and agreeing upon a signal the patient may give, either verbal or nonverbal, should they need to signal distress during the exam. Allowing patients to ask questions about the exam prior to initiating physical contact is another way to help empower patients to feel in control of their body and their medical care [4].

Women with opioid use disorder often have physical findings that should be noted. Poor dentition is common in people with substance use disorders, and should not be ignored in pregnancy. Noting damaged or missing teeth, caries, or gingival disease should prompt a referral for dental care [5]. Cardiac murmurs or rubs may be present, as well as pulmonary findings such as wheezes, crackles, or increased expiratory phase. Cutaneous signs of injection use (intravenous, subcutaneous, or intramuscular) might include a range of findings, from mild bruising and scarring to necrosis of skin and soft tissue. Edema of hands or extremities may be noted due to vascular or lymphatic injury from injection. If the patient consents, a breast exam may reveal use of veins of the breast for injection use. Noting hepatomegaly or hepatic tenderness on exam would prompt further evaluation. The provider should also note any signs concerning for interpersonal violence, such as bruising, abrasions, ligature marks, or genital or anal injuries [6], and document such injuries in accordance with recommendations from the National Institute of Justice. Even if the patient does not wish to file a police report about any abuse she is experiencing at that point in time, a clear and comprehensive medical record, including photographs of injuries if appropriate and patient consents, can provide helpful evidence should the abuse ever be reported or prosecuted [7].

## Infectious Disease

One of the most commonly recognized and variable health consequences for women with opioid use disorder in pregnancy is infection. Risk for infection comes not only from the substance use itself, especially injection use, but also from sexual practices or partners with high prevalence of infectious disease and/or limited access to harm reduction programs including syringe exchange [8]. People with substance use disorders also often have reduced immune function, nutritional deficiencies, and health complications from chronic stress and inadequate sleep, particularly salient for people also experiencing intermittent or chronic homelessness (Figure 7.1).

## Sexually Transmitted Disease

### GC/CT/Trichomonas/HSV/HPV/Syphilis

Providing care to pregnant women with opiate use disorder provides the opportunity for a complete

| Cardiovascular | Infectious endocarditis<br>Thromboembolic disease<br>Heart failure<br>Phlebitis |
| --- | --- |
| Pulmonary | Asthma<br>Pneumonitis<br>Thermal inhalant injury<br>Granulomatous disease |
| Gastrointestinal | Chronic nausea<br>Delayed gastric emptying<br>Opioid-induced constipation |
| Endocrinopathies | Oligomenorrhea<br>Amenorrhea<br>Osteopenia<br>Osteoporosis |
| Soft tissue and bone infection | Cellulitis<br>Abscess<br>Vasculitis<br>Skin ulceration<br>Necrotizing fasciitis<br>Osteomyelitis |

**Figure 7.1** Additional medical complications associated with opiate use disorder [9–12]

evaluation of and, if necessary, treatment for sexually transmitted illness. Some women with opiate use disorder are at increased risk for STI, especially if they have been involved in work in the sex trade. Women with substance use disorder in general are at higher risk than the general population for sexual assault, coerced sex, sex with multiple partners, and other risky sexual behaviors. Women with injection drug use in particular have been shown to have lower rates of use of condoms, higher rates of multiple sexual partners, and higher rates of undetected or untreated STIs [13]. Providing testing and treatment for STIs, screening for cervical cancer, and potentially providing vaccination for HPV (human papilloma virus) after delivery can have long-reaching health impact for this patient population, as well as opportunity to increase sexual health literacy and self-efficacy [14].

## Viral Hepatitis

### Hepatitis B

Hepatitis B (HBV) is estimated to impact approximately 0.7–0.9 percent of pregnant women in the United States, with more than 25,000 infants at risk per year of vertical transmission leading to chronic HBV infection [15, 16]. Vertical transmission from mother to child remains a major source of perpetuation of chronic HBV worldwide. Given this high risk for vertical transmission, as well as effective available treatments to reduce risk of transmission, it has been recommended for several years that all pregnant women be screened for Hepatitis B in pregnancy with a test of hepatitis B surface antigen (HBsAg). Testing for HBV surface antibody alone does not rule chronic infection in or out, and thus HBsAg testing is the preferred assessment [17].

Relevant to the population of pregnant women with opiate use disorder, women who are at risk for Hepatitis B infection (>1 sexual partner during last 6 months, evaluated or treated for a sexually transmitted disease, history of or current injection substance use, or a sexual partner with known positive HBsAg) and do not have demonstrated immunity to HBV should be offered immunization.

For many women, chronic HBV may be asymptomatic, and thus screening in pregnancy may lead to their initial diagnosis of HBV. For these women, antenatal counseling is crucial, as there are approved treatments for both mother and neonate to help prevent vertical transmission.

Given that exposure to blood and body fluids is one major risk for transmission of HBV, there has been some debate about the safety of invasive antenatal testing (chorionic villous sampling or amniocentesis). Current guidelines recommend that for women with an indication for genetic testing with an invasive procedure, appropriate counseling for women with HBV RNA viral load >7 log 10 copies/mL should include a possible increased risk for maternal–fetal transmission. At time of delivery, invasive labor procedures such as internal monitors or operative vaginal delivery should not be prevented if indicated. This increased risk of transmission by exposure through either invasive prenatal or intranatal procedures is not thought to be greater than the protection conferred by perinatal infection prevention with both passive and active immunization given to exposed infants. Similarly, planned cesarean section is not recommended for the sole indication of attempt to reduce maternal–fetal transmission of HBV [16].

The significant advances in reducing maternal–fetal transmission of HBV have traditionally centered on providing passive and active immunity to HBV to the exposed infant within 12 hours from birth. By providing the combination of HBV immunoglobulin and HBV vaccine, it has been shown that durable protection from chronic HBV can be provided to 85–95 percent of exposed infants. Current recommendations are to provide this combination of passive and active immunity to all HBV exposed infants, including infants whose mother's HBsAg status is unknown. For infants who receive prophylaxis, breastfeeding is recommended.

As more recent evidence has demonstrated benefit for antenatal viremia reduction in prevention of vertical transmission of HBV, antiviral therapy has been increasingly offered to appropriate pregnant candidates. Since maternal viral load has been shown to be a direct indicator of immunoprophylaxis failure, checking HBV RNA viral load at time of initial diagnosis and in the third trimester is now recommended. In pregnant women with HBV viral load greater than 6–8 log 10 copies/mL, HBV antiviral therapy should be considered for the purpose of decreasing maternal viral load and thus reducing risk of vertical transmission. Referral to maternal–fetal medicine, hepatology, or infectious disease practitioners with experience treating HBV in pregnancy is appropriate at time of diagnosis, or in the third trimester for consideration of antiviral therapy, and for continued coordinated care and surveillance for women after delivery (Figure 7.2).

## Hepatitis C

As the opioid epidemic has reached critical importance in the public health, and more broadly, societal eye, so too has the increase in rates of Hepatitis C (HCV). Historically, screening tests for Hepatitis C have been

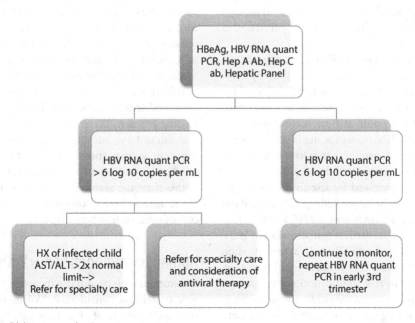

**Figure 7.2** Hepatitis B laboratory evaluation

Currently accepted risk factors:
Current injection drug use
History of injection drug use
Blood transfusion before 1992
Hemodialysis
HIV infection
Birth year between 1945–1965

Consider screening:
History of drug use by route other than injection
History of multiple sexual partners
History of working in sex trade
History of incarceration
History of body piercing or tattoo
Personal history or partner with STI
History of partner with HCV
Patient's mother with HCV

**Figure 7.3** Hepatitis C screening [19, 21]

offered to patients with identifiable risk factors, such as known injection substance use. Other identified risk factors for HCV that have been broadly accepted are blood transfusion or products, organ transplantation prior to 1992, hemodialysis, or HIV coinfection. Testing women with these identifiable risks in pregnancy is recommended by both the Centers for Disease Control and Prevention and the American College of Obstetrics and Gynecologists, but universal screening in pregnancy has not been considered a cost-effective strategy [18]. However, as newer research has demonstrated, using a policy of testing for HCV in only women with such identifiable risk factors has significant limitations, such that between 28 and 40 percent of pregnant women with HCV could go unidentified (Figure 7.3) [19, 20].

If a woman with opioid use disorder is offered testing, and does in fact test positive for HCV, many laboratories will now reflexively test for HCV RNA viral load as well as genotype. Testing hepatic function studies at the same time would also be recommended. If this type of reflexive laboratory testing is not in place, a positive HCV antibody would then necessitate further testing as mentioned above. While no antiviral therapies have been yet approved for use in the treatment of HCV in pregnancy or breastfeeding, this should not discourage providers from testing for HCV in the antenatal period. Given that vertical transmission of HCV is estimated at 2–10 percent [22], vertical transmission remains one of the most common routes of infection, and is comparable in risk to injection substance use. Providing appropriate antenatal guidance for the pregnant woman regarding vertical transmission rates and

neonatal follow up should be included as part of the care for our pregnant patients with opiate use disorder and HCV. Patients should also be educated that unless they have HIV co-infection, HCV is not a contraindication to breastfeeding. Also of note, pregnancy is not a contraindication to Hepatitis B vaccination, and should be offered to any pregnant woman with HCV who is not immune to Hepatitis B. Safety of the Hepatitis A (HAV) vaccine in pregnancy has not been determined; although, given that HAV vaccine is produced from inactivated HAV, the theoretical risk to the fetus would be expected to be low [23].

As mentioned above, to date there is no approved antiviral therapy for pregnant or breastfeeding women with HCV; however, some animal model data has suggested that there may be safety data for antiviral treatment in pregnancy. The impact of maternal viremia level as it relates to risk for vertical transmission of HCV is not well-defined, but reports of mothers with undetectable HCV RNA levels reveal rare transmission. Using other infectious disease models, such as HBV and HIV, which clearly demonstrate risk reduction of vertical transmission with maternal viral load reduction, it seems reasonable that a decrease in viremia in pregnant women with HCV would thus reduce risk of vertical transmission. While we await further safety data regarding use of antiviral therapy for pregnant women with HCV, more research is being conducted currently on an observational level to determine at which threshold of viremia below which vertical transmission does not occur, and whether planned cesarean section prevents mother-to-child transmission (Eunice Kennedy Shriver National Institute of Child Health and Development Maternal Fetal Medicine Units Network) [21]. While currently there remain more questions than answers regarding evaluation and treatment of HCV in pregnant and breastfeeding women, there is hope that ongoing research and safety trials might one day make treatment for pregnant women a possibility. We should also continue to educate our patients that HCV is not an indication at this time for planned cesarean section, and nor is HCV, unless there is known co-infection with HIV, a contraindication to breastfeeding.

## Human Immunodeficiency Virus

For women with opioid use disorder, the risk of exposure to HIV is considerable. Women with injection substance use are at risk from sharing of needles, as well as sexual exposure from partners with unknown serostatus for HIV. Women with opioid use disorder, injection substance use, and working in the sex trade are among the highest risk for HIV exposure. Given that approximately 1 in 8 people living in the United States with HIV are unaware of their status [24], testing for HIV in pregnancy as per routine obstetric care will undoubtedly result in new diagnoses of HIV for women with opioid use disorder presenting for prenatal care.

When screening for HIV, the 4th generation antibody–antigen test is preferred. For women who test positive, confirmatory testing should be completed. For confirmed new diagnosis of HIV in pregnancy, additional testing is required as well as referral to specialty care (maternal-fetal medicine and/or infectious disease with experience treating women with HIV in pregnancy). At initial time of diagnosis, this additional testing should include CD 4 count, HIV RNA level, HAV, HBV, HCV, TB, CBC, CMP, and syphilis. Women should also receive or be referred for resistance testing for antiretroviral therapy. Women should be assessed for need for prophylaxis against opportunistic infection, following current HIV treatment guidelines [24]. Best practice also includes screening for interpartner violence and/or need for referral of patient's partner for testing or treatment. Assessing for need for immunization should also be completed: HAV, HBV, influenza, pneumococcus, HPV, and Tdap are all recommended for HIV positive women without documented immunity or recent immunization. A dating ultrasound should also be completed as early as possible in pregnancy to aid in planning for timing and route of delivery later in pregnancy [25–27].

Although the routes of vertical transmission of HIV in pregnancy are not perfectly understood, there does appear to be increased risk for transmission in labor and delivery. One proposed mechanism is maternal–fetal microtransfusion across the placenta, especially during uterine contractions. Another exposure risk during delivery includes exposure to maternal genital secretions and blood during vaginal delivery [28, 26]. There is also significant data to support that risk of vertical transmission of HIV is directly related to concentration of HIV RNA in maternal plasma, referred to as the viral load. For women with HIV and a viral load of less than 1,000 copies per mL, the risk for vertical transmission is as low at 2 percent [25, 26, 29].

The treatment of HIV in pregnancy is targeted at improving maternal health, but also reducing risk of

| |
|---|
| Diagnosis of STI during current pregnancy |
| Illicit drug use during current pregnancy |
| Exchange of sex for money or drugs |
| Multiple sex partners during current pregnancy |
| Signs/symptoms of acute HIV during pregnancy |
| Living in region with increased incidence of HIV in childbearing women |
| Partner with known HIV-positive serostatus |

**Figure 7.4** Indications for repeat HIV testing in 3rd trimester

vertical transmission to the fetus. Early treatment for pregnant women with HIV consisted of intrapartum zidovudine (ZDV) plus postexposure prophylaxis of the newborn for 6 weeks after birth. This treatment resulted in a significant reduction in vertical transmission rates of HIV, from greater than 25 percent with no care to 8 percent with ZVD and postexposure prophylaxis for the neonate. With the advent of combination therapy and antiretroviral therapy (ART), there are more options for targeted treatment to maximize both maternal and fetal wellbeing [26, 30].

Current recommendations are to begin ART as early as possible in pregnancy. Treatment should then be modified based on resistance testing results, but ART should not be delayed until this testing is complete. Early initiation of ART recognizes the need to reduce maternal HIV viral load to as low as possible, with the goal of viral load being undetectable. As most ART regimens take between 12 and 24 weeks for complete viral suppression, initiation of ART as early as possible gives the best opportunity for complete viral suppression by time of delivery. Current guideline recommendations for monitoring of HIV viral load include at baseline, 2–4 weeks after initiation or change in ART, monthly until RNA is undetectable, and then every 3 months through the remainder of pregnancy. A viral load should also be checked between 34 and 36 weeks to assist patient and provider shared decision making regarding timing and mode of delivery (Figure 7.4) [25–27, 29, 31].

Mode of delivery requires careful shared decision making between patient and her obstetrics provider. Current guideline recommendations use an RNA level of 1,000 copies per mL as a decision point for mode of delivery. For women with undetectable viral load or less than 1,000 copies per mL, there remains a vertical transmission rate of approximately 2 percent, which has not been shown to be increased by vaginal delivery. For women with viral load greater than 1,000 copies per mL, the recommendation is for planned cesarean delivery before the onset of labor or rupture of membranes (ROM). To increase the likelihood for delivery prior to onset of labor or ROM, many recommend delivery by planned cesarean section at 38 weeks gestation. This conversation between patient and provider must also include the information that no medication or mode of delivery has been able to reduce risk of vertical transmission to zero [27, 32].

For women who are HIV positive, even on ART, the recommendation remains to avoid breastfeeding to prevent neonate exposure to HIV in breast milk.

Part of care for pregnant women with HIV should also include counseling about the need for ongoing ART after delivery, as well as follow up for their infant, ideally with a pediatric HIV specialist. Care for a pregnant woman's partner should also include referral for testing and potentially preexposure prophylaxis (PrEP) if appropriate [32]. This type of coordinated care has been shown to increase adherence to ART, thereby providing the best possible outcomes for women, infants, and their families.

## Opioid Dependence in the Setting of Chronic Pain

Special comment needs to be made regarding a subgroup of women with opioid use in pregnancy: women with chronic pain treated with chronic opioid therapy (COT). This group of patients is heterogeneous with respect to pain etiologies but the commonality of opioid dependence (defined as physiological adaptation to opioid medication such that sudden cessation of medication precipitates expected, class-specific withdrawal symptoms) presents a unique concern in pregnancy. Given that women are prescribed more opioids than men [33], and at higher doses and for longer periods of time [34], treatment concerns for these women who become pregnant continue to grow.

A pregnant woman presenting with opioid dependence in the setting of COT presents an opportunity for shared decision making regarding her medication and treatment. The first determination should be whether a patient with opioid dependence also has features of opioid use disorder. These women would most appropriately be cared for with referral for further assessment and treatment, and should be considered for MAT (medication assisted treatment).

For women who present without features of opioid use disorder, but do have physiologic dependence, treatment goals should be determined together. Some patients, even with moderate to severe chronic pain conditions, will be motivated to taper their medication during pregnancy given the risk of neonatal abstinence syndrome (NAS) as well as concern about ability to breastfeed safely. Some women have the goal of discontinuing COT completely in pregnancy. These patients with opioid dependence who desire to discontinue or taper their medications present prenatal providers with a unique opportunity to decrease medication burden and risks of chronic opioid exposure, but one rarely taken given the historical concerns about discontinuing opioids in pregnancy.

Historically, detoxification from opioids in pregnancy was discouraged based largely on two influential reports published in the 1970s. The first, a report by Rementeria and Nuang [35], described a pregnant woman with heroin use, who had a term fetal demise in the setting of severe opiate withdrawal. The second report, by Zuspan et al. [36], described elevated amine (epinephrine and norepinephrine) in the amniotic fluid of a woman undergoing a methadone taper. These two cases, published within 2 years of one another, had a profound impact on the prenatal medical community, and resulted in a fear of opioid detoxification in pregnancy.

Since those reports in the 1970s, there have been periodic reports of detoxification from opioids in pregnancy with more encouraging maternal and neonatal outcomes. Several publications describe detoxification from opiates in all trimesters of pregnancy, without increased incidence of miscarriage, preterm delivery, or stillbirth compared to control population [37–40]. However, detoxification is different from a slow, methodical outpatient taper. Detoxification, even in the studies with the longest timeframes, is typically conducted over days to weeks, often in an inpatient facility; COT taper protocols typically occur over weeks to months [41, 42] and are outpatient. For pregnant women without opioid use disorder, it is increasingly accepted to slowly taper COT medications over weeks to months of pregnancy, with the goal of decreasing the risk for NAS, as well as improving the likelihood of being able to safely breastfeed.

In order to provide a safe and successful COT taper, provider and patient must be in agreement about goals. For some women, it will not be possible to significantly reduce or stop their opioid therapy. These women need to be counseled prior to delivery about pain control in labor, neonatal abstinence syndrome, and breastfeeding. For women who desire to taper opioids or stop opioid therapy completely during pregnancy, shared

**First Visit**

Assess for opioid dependence

Assess for opioid use disorder criteria

Calculate morphine milliequivalents (MME)

Urine toxicology, including opiate panel

Prescription drug monitoring database check

Shared decision making regarding goals for taper:

reduce MME, taper off, safely breastfeed, reduce risk of NAS

Controlled substance agreement provider–patient contract signed

Plan to reduce opioid dose by 5–10% MME per week

**Subsequent visits (recommend every 1–2 weeks)**

Calculate current MME

Urine toxicology

Prescription drug monitoring database check

Increase adjuvant pain treatment: physical therapy, massage, TENS unit, nonopioid medications, etc.

Mental health support: counseling, groups, psychoeducation

Continue to refine goals and counsel regarding pain control in labor, NAS, and breastfeeding

Continue to reduce opioid dose by 5–10% MME every 1–2 weeks

**Figure 7.5** Suggested components of care for opioid tapering

goal setting is paramount. For providers with comfort prescribing and tapering opioids, this tapering may be done in the context of the patient's routine prenatal visits. For providers with limited experience with opioids prescribing, careful coordination between prenatal care provider and pain specialist is essential. The following illustration provides a sample of the elements useful in tapering patients off chronic opioid therapy (Figure 7.5).

# References

1. Chitwood D. D., Sanchez J., Comerford M., McCoy C. B. Primary preventative health care among injection drug users, other sustained drug users, and nonusers. *Subst Use Misuse* 2001 May–June; 36(6–7):807–24.

2. Chitwood D. D., McBride D. C., French M. T., Comerford M. Health care need and utilization: A preliminary comparison of injection drug users, other illicit drug users, and nonusers. *Subst Use Misuse* 1999 Mar–Apr; 34(4–5):727–46.

3. Herron A. J., Brennan T. K. *The ASAM Essentials of Addiction Medicine*. Philadelphia, PA: Wolters Kluwer and American Society of Addiction Medicine; 2015.

4. Raja S., Hasnain M., Hoersch M., Gove-Yin S., Raiagopalan C. Trauma informed care in medicine: current knowledge and future research. *Fam Community Health* 2015; 38(2):216–26.

5. Shekarchizadeh H., Khami M. R., Mohebbi S. Z., Ekhtiari H., Virtanen J. I. Oral health of drug abusers: a review of health effects and care. *Iran J Public Health* 2013; 42(9):929–40.

6. Kramer A., Lorenzon D., Mueller G. Prevalence of intimate partner violence and health implications for women using emergency departments and primary care clinics. *Womens Health Issues* 2004; 14(1):19–29.

7. Isaac N. E., Pualani Enos V. *Documenting Domestic Violence: How Health Care Providers Can Help Victims*. National Institute of Justice Research in Brief. September 2001.

8. Gibson D. R., Flynn N. M., Perales D. Effectiveness of syringe exchange program in reducing HIV risk behavior and HIV seroconversion among injecting drug users. *AIDS* 2001; 15:1329–41.

9. Wurcel A. G., Merchant E. A., Clark R. P., Stone D. R. Emerging and underrecognized complications of illicit drug use. Goldstein EJC, ed. *Clinical Infectious Diseases: An Official Publication of the Infectious Diseases Society of America*. 2015; 61(12):1840–9. doi: 10.1093/cid/civ689.

10. Connolly C., O'Donoghue K., Doran H., McCarthy F. P. Infective endocarditis in pregnancy: Case report and review of the literature. *Obstet Med* 2015; 8(2):102–4.

11. Wolff A. J., O'Donnell A. E. Pulmonary effects of illicit drug use. *Clin Chest Med* 2004 Mar; 25(1):203–16.

12. Mégarbane B., Chevillard L. The large spectrum of pulmonary complications following illicit drug use: features and mechanisms. *Chem Biol Interact* 2013 Dec 5; 206(3):444–51.

13. Centers for Disease Control and Prevention (2013) *HIV in the United States: At a Glance*. Available at: www.cdc.gov/hiv/pdf/statistics_basics_factsheet.pdf. Retrieved November 20, 2016.

14. Tyndall M. W., Patrick D., Spittal P., Li K., O'Shaughnessy M. V. Risky sexual behaviors among injection drug users with high HIV prevalence: implications for STD control. *Sex Transm Infect* 2002; 78(Suppl 1):i170–5.

15. Salemi J. L., Spooner K. K., Meija de Grubb M. C., et al. National trends of Hepatitis B and C during pregnancy across sociodemographic, behavioral, and clinical factors, United States, 1998–2011. *J Med Virol* 2017; 89(6):1025–32. Wiley Online Library. Retrieved December 3, 2016.

16. Dionne-Odom J., Tita A. T., Silverman N. S. Hepatitis B in pregnancy screening, treatment, and prevention of vertical transmission. *Am J Obstet Gynecol* 2016; 214(1):6–14.

17. Lin K., Vickery J. Screening for hepatitis B virus infection in pregnant women: evidence for the US Preventative Task For reaffirmation recommendation statement. *Ann Intern Med* 2009; 150:874–6.

18. Pergam S. A., Wang C. C., Gardella C. M., et al. Pregnancy complications associate with hepatitis C: data from a 2003–2005 Washington state birth cohort. *Am J Obstet Gynecol* 2008; 199:38.

19. Fernandez N., Towers C. V., Wolf L., et al. Sharing of snorting straws and hepatitis C infection in pregnant women. *Obstet Gynecol* 2016; 128:234–7.

20. Conte D., Fraquelli M., Prati D., et al. Prevalence and clinical course of chronic hepatitis C virus (HCV) infection and rate of HCV vertical transmission in a cohort of 15,250 pregnant women. *Hepatology* 2000; 31:751–5.

21. Prasad M. R. Hepatitis C virus screening in pregnancy: Is it time to change our practice? *Am Coll Obstet Gynecol* 2016; 128(2):229–30.

22. Kanninen T. T., Dieterich D., Asciutti S. HCV vertical transmission in pregnancy: New horizons in the era of DAAs. *Hepatology* 2015; 62:1656–8.

23. Centers for Disease Control and Prevention. *Guidelines for Vaccinating Pregnant Women, Hepatitis A*. 2014. Available at: www.cdc.gov/vaccines/pubs/preg-guide.htm#hepa. Retrieved August 31, 2016.

24. Centers for Disease Control and Prevention. *HIV Basics*. Available at: www.cdc.gov/hiv/basics/statistics .html. Retrieved December 4 2016.

25. Centers for Disease Control and Prevention. Report of the NIH Panel to define principles of therapy of HIV infection and guidelines for the use of antiretroviral agents in HIV-infected adults and adolescents. *MMWR Morb Wkly Rep* 1998; 47(RR-5):1–82.

26. Mofeson L. M., Lambert J. S., Stiehm E. R., et al. Risk factors for perinatal transmission of human immunodeficiency virus type 1 treated with zidovudine. Pediatric AIDS Clinical Trials Group Study 185 Team. *N Engl J Med* 1999; 341:385–93.

27. ACOG Committee Opinion Scheduled Cesarean Delivery and the Prevention of Vertical Transmission of HIV Infection. May 2000. Number 234.

28. Connor E. M., Perling R. S., Gelber R., et al. Reduction of maternal-infant transmission of human immunodeficiency virus type 1 with zidovudine treatment. Pediatric AIDS Clinical Trials Group Protocol 076 Study Group. *N Engl J Med* 1994; 331:1173–80.

29. Garcia P. M., Kalish L. A., Pitts J., et al. Maternal levels of plasma human immunodeficiency virus type 1 RNA and the risk of perinatal transmission. Women and Infants Transmission Study Group. *N Engl J Med* 1999; 341:349–402.

30. Panel on Treatment of HIV-Infected Pregnant Women and Prevention of Perinatal Transmission. Recommendations for Use of Antiretroviral Drugs in Pregnant HIV-1-Infected Women for Maternal Health and Interventions to Reduce Perinatal HIV Transmission in the United States. Available at: http://aidsinfo.nih.gov/contentfiles/lvguidelines/PerinatalGL.pdf. Retrieved February 01, 2017.

31. Seigfried N., van der Merwe L., Brocklehurst P., Sint T. T. Antiretrovirals for reducing the risk of mother-to-child transmission of HIV infection. *Cochrane Database Syst Rev* 2011; (7): Art. No.: CD003510.

32. Sebitloane H. M., Moodley D. The impact of highly active antiretroviral therapy on obstetric conditions: A review. *Eur J Obstet Gynecol Reprod Biol* 2017; 210:126–31.

33. Green T. C., Grimes-Serrano J. M., Licari A., Budman S. H., Butler S. F. Women who abuse prescription opioids: Findings from the Addiction Severity Index-Multimedia Version Connect prescription opioid database. *Drug Alcohol Depend* 2009; 103:65–73.

34. Cicero T. J., Wong G., Tian Y., et al. Co-morbidity and utilization of medical services by pain patients receiving opioid medications: Data from an insurance claims database. *Pain* 2009; 144:20–7.

35. Rementeria J. L., Nuang N. N. Narcotic withdrawal in pregnancy: Stillbirth incident with a case report. *Am J Obstet Gynecol* 1973; 116:1152–6.

36. Zuspan F. P., Gumpel J. A., Meija-Zelaya A., Madden J., Davis R. Fetal stress from methadone withdrawal. *Am J Obstet Gynecol* 1975; 122:43–6.

37. Stewart R. D., Nelson D. B., Adhikari E. H., et al. The obstetrical and neonatal impact of maternal opioid detoxification in pregnancy. *Am J Obstet Gynecol* 2013; 209:267. e1–5.

38. Dashe J. S., Sheffield J. S., Olschler D. A., Zane E. H., Wendel G. D. Opioid detoxification in pregnancy. *Obstet Gynecol* 1998; 92:854–8.

39. Bell J., Towers C. V., Henessy M. D., et al. Detoxification from opiate drugs during pregnancy. *Am J Obstet Gynecol* 2016; 215:374.e1–6.

40. Luty J., Nikolaou V., Bearn J. Is opiate detoxification unsafe in pregnancy? *J Subst Abuse Tret* 2004; 24: 363–7.

41. Sullivan M. D., Turner J. A., DiLodovico C., et al. Prescription opioid taper support for outpatients with chronic pain: a randomized controlled trial. *J Pain* 2016;10: 1–25.

42. Fiellen D. A., Schottenfeld M. D., Cutter C. J., et al. Primary care-based buprenorphine taper vs maintenance therapy for prescription opioid dependence. *JAMA Intern Med* 2014; 174(12): 1947–54.

# 8

# Harm Reduction Principles in Women with Opioid Use Disorder in Pregnancy

Lauren Owens and Mishka Terplan

## What does Harm Reduction Mean?

Harm reduction refers to policies, program and practices that aim to reduce the harms associated with the use of psychoactive drugs in people unable or unwilling to stop. The defining features are the focus on the prevention of harm, rather than on the prevention of drug use itself, and the focus on people who continue to use drugs. [1]

The harm reduction movement emerged from the work primarily of activists but also health workers who, in the 1960s and 1970s, opposed the increasing criminalization of drug use and drug users [2]. In contradistinction to the dominant popular narrative of drugs as a danger to society, their work focused on the amelioration of risks at the level of the individual consumer. Parallel to this was the emergence of epidemiologic research on drugs, particularly alcohol. A 1976 analysis of drinking patterns among men following treatment for alcohol use disorder found that the majority returned to controlled drinking without the negative consequences that compelled their initial treatment [3]. These findings were met with resistance as they problematized the assumption of abstinence, the goal of alcohol treatment. These two threads combined in the response public health crisis of HIV/AIDS in the 1980s (specifically in the Netherlands and Great Britain) where the recognition of the failure of existing, abstinence-based models of care led to a more productive approach to substance use disorder treatment: harm reduction [4].

Almost every human society has used psychoactive substances as part of their cultural practice; however, addiction and its negative consequences is a more recent and modern development [5]. Prioritizing abstinence, an approach that may ignore psychosocial contributors to substance use, may be counterproductive [4], and can lead to penalizing people who use drugs [3]. In contrast, proponents of harm reduction accept that the use of alcohol and other drugs is part of society and that individuals have a multiplicity of reasons for use. Harm reduction rests upon the principle that care should be nonjudgmental and noncoercive and begin with an acceptance of people at their individual state of change. This includes abstinence as a possibility but not as a prerequisite for accessing services or the sole goal of care [6]. Traditional examples of harm reduction strategies include syringe exchange, overdose training and naloxone dispensing, and safe injection facilities. However, any approach that prioritizes the needs of the patient and meets them where they are, such as condoms, contraception, and pre- (and post-) exposure prophylaxis for HIV, should also be considered harm reduction.

The beneficiaries of harm reduction are not just people directly involved in programs [7]. Syringe exchange programs are not only cost effective in terms of savings in cases of HIV prevented, but safe disposal of syringes also minimizes the risk of needle-stick injuries from improperly disposed of syringes in the community. Additionally, harm reduction benefits not just people with addiction, but anyone who uses drugs or alcohol [8]. Key features of harm reduction programs include utilizing client desires to shape the programs, lowering thresholds to services, reducing stigma, working to mitigate effects of more than one high-risk behavior, and providing multifaceted services to address more than just substance use and its consequences [9].

Key characteristics of harm reduction services:

- Nonjudgmental and noncoercive
- Low threshold
- Multiple points of entry
- Located in areas convenient to clients
- Collaborative program and individual goals
- Holistic services
- Client-staff relationships lack strict hierarchy
- Anonymous services (when possible and if desired)

## Harm Reduction as a Response to the War on Drugs

A nation's value system and treatment of persons who violate the norms are closely intertwined. [10]

Since 1971, the primary response to drug use and addiction in the United States has been through the so-called War on Drugs, a policy that has been termed "harm induction" as it promotes criminalization over counseling for people who use drugs [10]. Indeed, federal drug control spending has continued to emphasize enforcement, prosecution and incarceration domestically, and interdiction, eradication, and military escalation abroad although investments in treatment reduce crime and are more cost-effective [11, 12].

Criminalization of illicit substance use leads to disenfranchisement, overutilization of custody for nonviolent offenders, and repercussions such as exclusion from public housing [13]. The emphasis on criminalization in the United States led to a 10-fold increase in incarceration for drug-related offenses between 1980 and 1990 without any decrease in addiction or substance-related problems in society – a time frame in which both emergency room visits for issues related to substance use and incidence of HIV and hepatitis among people who inject drugs rose as well [14]. Abstinence-related prevention approaches, particularly the D.A.R.E., a program for school-aged children, have demonstrated similar lack of effectiveness; a meta-analysis of D.A.R.E. programs did not show lasting positive effects [15]. Despite its ineffectiveness, D.A.R.E. has enjoyed more positive publicity and support than syringe exchange programs [16]. Pregnant women who use drugs have also been specific targets of "harm inducing" policies. In 2014, for example, Tennessee passed a law allowing for the criminal prosecuting of pregnant women who use drugs for exposure and, if they suffered a miscarriage, they could be prosecuted for homicide as well [17]. Rather than decreasing substance use, this law led to women avoiding prenatal care, presenting late to prenatal care, delivering across state lines, and delivering at home [18]. Due in part to the fact that neonatal abstinence rates did not decrease, the law was allowed to sunset in 2016.

## Harm Reduction in the Context of Treatment for Pregnant Women

Based on experience since 1985, the rhetorical and policy-oriented emphasis on making drug use less acceptable and drugs less available, as well as the focus on drug prevalence as the dominant indicator of program success, has probably outlived its usefulness. [14]

People who use drugs are subject to great societal inequalities and burdens: poverty, trauma, racism, stigma associated with mental health condition, and other inequities. Moreover, the stigmatization of addiction, which is even stronger among pregnant women than the population at large, can drive people who use drugs away from treatment and other services [19]. People with other recognized medical issues such as cancer or heart disease benefit from organized, publicized non-profits that contribute to research and amelioration of suffering secondary to these illnesses. However, given the stigma associated with drug use, there are fewer advocacy organizations for people with addiction [9].

Women who use drugs, particularly in pregnancy, are more stigmatized and experience greater discrimination than other women and men with addiction [20]. Society and the law disproportionately target and penalize these women often under the banner of fetal protection and at the expense of the woman's human rights [21]. Such actions are barriers to initiating and continuing prenatal care [22, 23]. Women who use drugs may also hesitate to seek care for fear that their children will be removed from their care [24] and may be pressured to have abortions [22].

Holistic and harm reduction approaches to service for women with opioid use disorder, particularly those who already have children, may lead to improved outcomes for women and their children. A synthesis of qualitative literature found that involving children in women's recovery programs was associated with better motor, social, and language skills for the children. For the mothers, confidence in parenting and parenting skills increased, leading to more positive interactions with their children [25]. Pregnancy and birth among women who use drugs must be normalized. Instead of treating care episodes as opportunities for crisis intervention (thereby reinforcing stigma and bias), women should be safe to disclose and discuss their substance use without fearing it will jeopardize their access to care, take away their ability to parent, or result in their incarceration [4].

There are many ways to lower the barriers to services for pregnant women who use drugs: eliminating abstinence as a prerequisite for services; creating mobile services; and utilizing input from clients to tailor services to their expressed needs, not providers' perceptions of clients' needs. When services are run or designed by people who use or used to use drugs, the balance of power between providers and clients becomes more equal, stigma is reduced, and clients are empowered. Using harm reduction services to address multiple facets of clients' lives allows for the focus to be not just on drug use, but on other priorities expressed by clients: housing, food, health care, and relationships with family, for example [26].

Peer services are important to consider in treatment programming for pregnant women who use drugs. Peers can serve not only as patient-navigators, but can role-model healthy behavior as well [27]. Compared with professional staff, peers were better able to reduce inpatient use and improve recovery outcomes among individuals with serious mental illness [28]. Additionally, peer service programs provide workforce opportunities for women in recovery who may not have the education or work experience for many jobs.

## Examples of Harm Reduction for Women with Opioid Use Disorders in Pregnancy

We have come to recognize that double standards of morality, reproduction, and mothering, as well as legal and social inequality, shape women's experience. Because women have the capacity to become pregnant, they have been judged and regulated differently than men. [4]

## Syringe Exchange Programs

In response to a pharmacy's refusal to sell injection equipment to people who injected drugs in Amsterdam, syringe exchange programs (SEPs) were developed in the early 1980s [16]. These SEPs were sponsored by governments in collaboration with private organizations of people who injected drugs. The first syringe exchange in the United States was implemented in Tacoma, Washington, in 1988 [29]. In one study, HIV incidence in people who inject drugs dropped by 6 percent per year in cities with SEPs and increased by 6 percent per year in cities without SEPs [30]. Since initiation of SEPs in Philadelphia, the percent of new HIV cases attributed to intravenous drug use dropped from 51 percent in 1992 to 17.5 percent in 2007 [8]. A cost estimate study incorporating SEPs, pharmacy sales, and syringe disposal programs found that each HIV infection averted would cost an

estimated $34,278; in comparison, the lifetime cost of treating HIV infection at the time of the publication (1998) was $108,649 [31].

The role of SEPs for pregnant women with opioid use disorder can be even more crucial. In addition to the individual level risk of HIV/HCV acquisition, pregnant women can transmit illness vertically – to the fetus/newborn at the time of delivery. Making SEPs accessible and friendly to pregnant women is crucial, both in terms of overcoming the added stigma of gender and pregnancy and in the additional harm reduction of serving pregnant women. One strategy to make programming more accessible for women is to have "ladies' nights." Dedicating services to people who identify as women-only is appreciated by participants, who see these as safe, empowering places [32].

Although many SEPs are in buildings, some SEPs are mobile, further reducing the threshold to services. A mobile SEP in Baltimore targets a section of town with multiple exotic dance clubs. A baseline survey performed as part of the mobile SEP's programming found that 75 percent of women seeking SEP services through the program were not accessing reproductive health services [33]. This program was established in 2008 and expanded to include reproductive health services in 2009 [34]. Through the mobile services, women access syringe exchange, pregnancy testing and options counseling, contraceptive counseling and methods, and vaccinations. Of women seeking injectable contraception through the mobile services, those seeking additional services (e.g. vaccines or emergency contraception) were more likely to continue that contraception [34]. This illustrates that making multiple services available in one location, particularly via outreach, can increase uptake of complementary services.

## Special Needs in Pregnancy Service

In the mid-1980s, Dr. Mary Hepburn established a clinic in Glasgow, Glasgow Women's Reproductive Health Services, to offer woman-centered care through a harm reduction approach. The clinic, now known as Special Needs in Pregnancy Service, offers prenatal care to women who use drugs, and has been a model for clinics elsewhere in Great Britain [4]. Providing help with nonmedical issues at Hepburn's clinic improved women's attendance at antenatal care [35]. The clinic utilizes social workers not just for crisis management, but for preventive assistance. Women can refer themselves to the clinic and be seen without a fee [35].

59

Pregnant women need not commit to either abstinence or opioid agonist maintenance to participate in programming at the clinic. Those who want to attempt detoxification are also supported, as are those who continue drug use. The program focuses on meeting women "where they are" with respect to their substance use. Thanks to Dr. Hepburn's work, the UK's maternity strategy recognizes that substance use and other poverty-related issues need to be addressed within routine prenatal care [23].

## Sheway

Located in the Downtown Eastside neighborhood of Vancouver, Sheway has provided support to pregnant women and women with children up to 18 months of age since 1993 [24, 36]. The program is linked to Fir Square, a hospital that has several antepartum and postpartum beds dedicated to women with substance use disorders seeking treatment [37]. The program offers multidisciplinary services: counseling, social work, nutrition, pediatric and obstetric care, and parenting support. The medical clinic offers drop-in hours, eliminating the barrier of scheduling a prenatal care appointment. Care is trauma-informed, meaning that it recognizes the violence clients have survived and continue to survive, and works to build trust with clients. As a large percentage of clients are First Nations, the program employs First Nations staff as cooks, community support workers, and community health nurses. The program has achieved a large decrease in the percentage of children born to women with substance use disorders who are removed from their mothers' care: from 100 percent in 1993 to 26 percent in 2012 [24].

## Naloxone and Overdose Prevention

Similar to opioid agonist therapy and supervised injection sites, naloxone provision to people who use drugs can decrease mortality associated with opioid overdose [38]. Naloxone is an opioid antagonist that can be administered by lay personnel, first responders, or other medical staff to reverse an opioid overdose. Naloxone may be administered subcutaneously, intramuscularly, intravenously, or intranasally. Repeated doses may be necessary depending on the strength and half-life of the inciting opioid. When administered intranasally, the half-life is 2 hours; via the other routes, the half-life is 0.5–1.5 hours [39]. Naloxone can be prescribed, dispensed, or handed out as part of public health outreach efforts.

Clinicians should offer naloxone to all people who use opioids, including those on chronic opioid therapy and those with treated and untreated addiction. Recent incarceration or admission for medically supervised withdrawal from opioids are risk factors for overdose as are a history of overdose and concurrent benzodiazepine or alcohol use. Overdose education and nasal naloxone should go to individuals meeting these criteria as well as friends and family – other potential overdose witnesses [40, 41]. State-specific policies vary; Prescribe to Prevent is a good and updated resource (http://prescribetoprevent.org/research-legal/legal/) [42].

Naloxone has been a successful tool in combating the overdose epidemic. During a 3-year follow-up of overdose education and nasal naloxone distribution programs in Massachusetts, naloxone was successful in reversing overdose in 98 percent of attempts (150/153) [38]. In communities implementing these programs, fatal overdose rates were 37–46 percent lower than that in communities not implementing the programs. A meta-analysis of overdose education and naloxone administration programs showed that naloxone administration by overdose witnesses was associated with a nearly 8-fold increased likelihood of overdose survival compared to no naloxone administration [43].

## Conclusions

In caring for pregnant women with opioid use disorder, we envision and advocate doing what can be done rather than focusing on what "should" be done. Pregnant women who use drugs are vulnerable to multiple factors that predispose them to adverse obstetrical outcomes, thus confounding any effect of substance use: low socioeconomic status, poor access to prenatal care, medical comorbidities, histories of trauma, and structural racism and stigma [4]. The intersection of womanhood, pregnancy, and opioid use is a place where harm reduction can profoundly improve care and change outcomes for a historically stigmatized, disenfranchised group. This begins by treating pregnant women who use drugs with dignity and respect.

## References

1. Harm Reduction International. *Home – Harm Reduction International.* Available at: www.hri.global/?no-splash=true. Retrieved January 7, 2017.
2. Roe G. Harm reduction as paradigm: Is better than bad good enough? The origins of harm reduction. *Crit Pub Health* 2005; 14(3):243–50.

3. David J. A., Polich J. M., Braiker H. B., *Alcoholism and Treatment*. Santa Monica, CA: Department of Health, Education, and Welfare. Available at: www.rand.org/pubs/reports/R1739.html. Retrieved January 22, 2017.

4. Boyd S., Marcellus L. *With Child: Substance Use During Pregnancy: A Woman-Centred Approach*. Ontario: Fernwood Publishing Company Limited; 2007.

5. Glasser I. *Anthropology of Addictions and Recovery*. Available at: www.amazon.com/Anthropology-Addictions-Recovery-Irene-Glasser/dp/1577665589%3FSubscriptionId%3DAKIAILSHYYTFIVPWUY6Q%26tag%3Dduckduckgo-ffab-20%26linkCode%3Dxm2%26camp%3D2025%26creative%3D165953%26creativeASIN%3D1577665589. Retrieved January 22, 2017.

6. Whittaker A. *Substance Misuse in Pregnancy*. Available at: www.drugsandalcohol.ie/20435/1/SubstanceMisusePregnancy.pdf. Retrieved January 30, 2017.

7. Newcombe R. The Reduction of Drug-Related Harm: A Conceptual Framework for Theory, Practice and Research. In: O'Hare P., editor. *The Reduction of Drug Related Harm*. London: Taylor & Francis Limited; 1992, pp. 1–15.

8. Evans A., White W., Lamb R. *The Role of Harm Reduction in Recovery-oriented Systems of Care: The Philadelphia Experience*. Available at: www.williamwhitepapers.com/pr/Recovery%20and%20Harm%20Reduction%20In%20Philadelphia.pdf. Retrieved January 5, 2017.

9. Marlatt G. Harm reduction: Come as you are. *Addict Behav* 1996; 21(6):779–88.

10. Wormer K. V. Harm induction vs harm reduction: Comparing American and British approaches to drug use. *J Offender Rehabil* 1999; 29(1–2):35–48.

11. Rydell C. Enforcement or treatment? Modeling the relative efficacy of alternatives for controlling cocaine. *Oper Res* 1996 Oct 1; 44(5):687–95.

12. Drug Policy Alliance. *The Federal Drug Control Budget: New Rhetoric, Same Failed Drug War*. Available at: www.drugpolicy.org/sites/default/files/DPA_Fact_sheet_Drug_War_Budget_Feb2015.pdf. Retrieved January 22, 2017.

13. Hunt N. *A Review of the Evidence Base for Harm Reduction Approaches to Drug Use*. Available at: www.hri.global/files/2010/05/31/HIVTop50Documents11.pdf. Retrieved January 8, 2017.

14. Reuter P., Caulkins J. P. Redefining the goals of national drug policy: Recommendations from a working group. *Am J Pub Health* 1995 Aug; 85(8 Pt 1):1059–63.

15. Ennett S. T., Tobler N. S., Ringwalt C. L., Flewelling R. L. How effective is drug abuse resistance education? A meta-analysis of Project DARE outcome evaluations. *Am J Pub Health* 1994; 84(9):1394–401.

16. Jarlais D. C. D., Sloboda Z., Friedman S. R., et al. Diffusion of the D.A.R.E. and syringe exchange programs. *Am J Pub Health* 2011; 96(8):1354–8.

17. Tate R., Weaver T. L. SB1391. Available at: www.capitol.tn.gov/Bills/108/Bill/SB1391.pdf. Retrieved January 30, 2017.

18. American Congress of Obstetricians and Gynecologists. *Support the Protecting Our Infants Act of 2015*. Available at: www.acog.org/-/media/Departments/Government-Relations-and-Outreach/2015ProtectingOurInfantsOnePager.pdf?dmc=1&ts=20170108T1743053530. Retrieved January 8, 2017.

19. Harm Reduction Coalition. *Getting off Right*. Available at: http://harmreduction.org/wp-content/uploads/2011/12/getting-off-right.pdf. Retrieved January 3, 2017.

20. Sales P., Murphy S. Surviving violence: Pregnancy and drug use. *J Drug Issues* 2000 Oct 1; 30(4):695–724.

21. Paltrow L. M., Flavin J. Arrests of and forced interventions on pregnant women in the United States, 1973–2005: Implications for women's legal status and public health. *J Health Polit Policy Law* 2013 Apr; 38(2):299–343.

22. Pinkham S., Myers B., Stoicescu C. Developing effective harm reduction services for women who inject drugs. In: Stoicescu C., editor. *The Global State of Harm Reduction: Towards an Integrated Response*. London: Harm Reduction International; 2012. p. 125–37.

23. Boyd S., Vukmirovich D. *Challenging Drug Prohibition & the Regulation of Reproduction and Mothering*. Available at: http://drugpolicy.ca/wp-content/uploads/2015/02/PUBLIC_FORUM_REPORT_Jan30.pdf. Retrieved January 30, 2017.

24. Revai T. *Sharing the Journey: The Sheway Model of Care*. Available at: http://sheway.vcn.bc.ca/files/2016/01/Sharing-the-Journey.pdf. Retrieved January 8, 2017.

25. Sword W., Jack S., Niccols A., et al. Integrated programs for women with substance use issues and their children: A qualitative meta-synthesis of processes and outcomes. *Harm Reduct J* 2009; 6:32.

26. Rogers S. J., Ruefli T. Does harm reduction programming make a difference in the lives of highly marginalized, at-risk drug users? *Harm Reduct J* 2004; 1:7.

27. Sherman B. R., Sanders L. M., Yearde J. Role-modeling healthy behavior: Peer counseling for pregnant and postpartum women in recovery. *Womens Health Issues Off Publ Jacobs Inst Womens Health* 1998 Aug; 8(4):230–8.

28. Chinman M., George P., Dougherty R. H., et al. Peer support services for individuals with serious mental illnesses: Assessing the evidence. *Psychiatr Serv Wash DC* 2014 Apr 1; 65(4):429–41.

29. Hagan H., Des Jarlais D. C., Purchase D., Reid T., Friedman S. R. The Tacoma syringe exchange. *J Addict Dis* 1991; 10(4):81–8.

30. Hurley S. F., Jolley D. J., Kaldor J. M. Effectiveness of needle-exchange programmes for prevention of HIV infection. *Lancet Lond Engl* 1997 Jun 21; 349(9068):1797–800.

31. Holtgrave D. R., Pinkerton S. D., Jones T. S., Lurie P., Vlahov D. Cost and cost-effectiveness of increasing access to sterile syringes and needles as an HIV prevention intervention in the United States. *J Acquir Immune Defic Syndr Hum Retrovirology Off Publ Int Retrovirology Assoc* 1998;18(Suppl 1):S133–8.

32. Magee C., Huriaux E. Ladies' night: Evaluating a drop-in programme for homeless and marginally housed women in San Francisco's mission district. *Int J Drug Policy* 2008 Apr; 19(2):113–21.

33. Moore E., Han J., Serio-Chapman C., et al. Contraception and clean needles: Feasibility of combining mobile reproductive health and needle exchange services for female exotic dancers. *Am J Pub Health* 2012 Oct; 102(10):1833–6.

34. Martin C. E., Han J. J., Serio-Chapman C., Chaulk P., Terplan M. Injectable contraceptive continuation among female exotic dancers seeking mobile reproductive health services. *J Health Care Poor Underserved* 2014 Aug; 25(3):1317–27.

35. Hepburn M. Drug use in pregnancy. *Br J Hosp Med* 1993; 49(1):51–5.

36. SHEWAY. *SHEWAY – A Community Project for Women and Children.* Available at: http://sheway.vcn.bc.ca/files/2012/05/sheway_brochure.pdf. Retrieved January 8, 2017.

37. BC Women's Hospital + Health Centre. *Pregnancy, Drugs & Alcohol.* Available at: www.bcwomens.ca/our-services/pregnancy-prenatal-care/pregnancy-drugs-alcohol. Retrieved January 8, 2017.

38. Walley A. Y., et al. Opioid overdose rates and implementation of overdose education and nasal naloxone distribution in Massachusetts: Interrupted time series analysis. *BMJ* 2013; 46:f174.

39. Lexicomp. Naloxone: Drug information. In: Post TW, editor, *UpToDate.* UpToDate, Waltham, MA. Accessed June 27, 2017.

40. Dowell D., Haegerich T. M., Chou R. CDC guideline for prescribing opioids for chronic pain – United States, 2016. *JAMA* 2016; 315(15):1624–45.

41. SAMHSA Opioid Overdose Toolkit. Available at: http://store.samhsa.gov/shin/content//SMA13-4742/Overdose_Toolkit_2014_Jan.pdf on 4/10/17.

42. Prescribe to Prevent. Available at: http://prescribetoprevent.org/research-legal/legal/. Retrieved June 27, 2017.

43. Giglio R. E., Li G., DiMaggio C. J. Effectiveness of bystander naloxone administration and overdose education programs: A meta-analysis. *InJ Epidemiol* 2015; 2(1):10.

Chapter

# 9

# Prenatal Care in Substance-Using Pregnant Women

Charles W. Schauberger

## Introduction

Pregnancy requires less than a year in the lifespan of a woman, but its impact on her future is enormous. Prenatal care is designed to guide women through pregnancy and to identify medical problems early and manage them successfully. All pregnant women can benefit from this care, but it is especially important for women with a history of substance use disorder (SUD).

Studies that demonstrate a close tie between receipt of prenatal care and improved outcomes in the typical pregnancy have been limited; however, a number of studies have found that the connection between prenatal care and resultant improved outcomes is strong for pregnant women with SUD. In a retrospective review from 1992, Broekhuizen et al. demonstrated that a minimum of 5 prenatal visits was associated with better outcomes in patients who used illicit drugs [1]. Berenson et al. found that having more than 3 prenatal visits was associated with better pregnancy outcomes for women using cocaine [2]. El-Mohandes et al. performed an extensive review of a Washington, DC, population in the mid-1990s and found that the highest rates of prematurity and low birthweight occurred in women who had no prenatal care and who used illicit drugs during pregnancy, and that these rates decreased as the number of prenatal care visits increased [3]. Although many of these studies suggest a dose–response curve between the number of prenatal visits and desired outcomes for pregnancy in women with SUD, the content or quality of the prenatal care these women received is largely unaddressed.

This chapter focuses on those elements of prenatal care that our experience suggests might require special attention in the pregnancies of women with SUD. Many elements of care remain constant, but the manner in which prenatal care is provided will differ greatly by circumstance. Not only do individual patient characteristics vary, but also the care women receive in resource-rich suburban settings is likely to be quite different from that provided in rural areas or in large inner-city settings. The literature offers scant support for the best practices suggested here, but they are offered to prompt discussion about how to maximize prenatal care in the office, clinic, or bedside. The goal is to provide the reader with tools that may assist in the care of women with these special considerations.

## Care Coordination

When care is provided by many individuals and for multiple conditions, there is a danger of missed care, contradictory recommendations, and suboptimal coordination caused by poor communication. All efforts must be made to prevent patients from being lost in a maze of appointments, meetings, and missed telephone calls. For many women with SUD, life is chaotic; pregnancy adds another level of complexity. It is paramount that the patient remains in the center of the care model (Figure 9.1).

For the obstetric care team and the addiction team, care coordination should occur at the first opportunity. In most pregnancies, the obstetrical care provider (obstetrician, family medicine provider, or nurse-midwife) serves as the coordinator of care. Training or experience in addiction care may vary, but either the obstetrical provider or an addiction provider must possess this competency. It is important to assess patient needs and who might best provide the necessary care. Who will prescribe which medications? Who will coordinate care to make sure she is not lost in the system? How will information be shared and with whom? It is important to have all the necessary release of information forms signed so all parties to the patient's care can communicate with each other.

Components of Quality Prenatal Care for Women with Substance Use Disorder

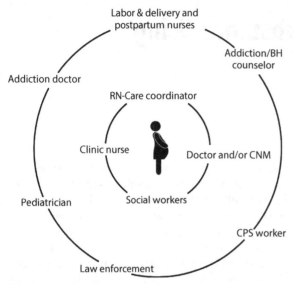

**Figure 9.1** Patient-centered model of care for pregnant women with SUD

# Early Pregnancy Considerations for Women with Substance Use Disorder

The rate of unplanned pregnancy is 50 percent for the general population [4, 5], but for patients with SUD, the rate may be as high as 85 percent [6]. Opioid use may affect ovulation, so irregular menses are more common in women who use them [7]. Contraception is used by approximately 50 percent of women with SUD. Many have a long history of unprotected intercourse without pregnancy [8], which leads them to believe that they could not conceive. Some early pregnancy symptoms may resemble withdrawal symptoms for some women, which further delays recognition of the pregnancy. Once they are sure they are pregnant, they may worry about how their pregnancy will be received by their partner, family, or treatment team. Some fear being pressured, or even forced, to terminate the pregnancy. Others worry that the pregnancy might require them to discontinue medically assisted treatment (MAT). An important aspect of early prenatal care is to address any patient concerns and expectations.

In our clinic, two-thirds of pregnant patients with SUD are already receiving addiction care when they arrive for their first prenatal visit. Many notify their methadone or buprenorphine clinic providers early in the pregnancy, and we prioritize early access for these patients in order to introduce them to prenatal care,

often before 8 weeks gestation. The other third of our patients are actively using drugs at their first prenatal visit and have had limited exposure to health care since childhood. They arrive at unpredictable durations of pregnancy and through multiple points of entry, including emergency services, county health departments, and jail medicine.

A positive pregnancy test may prompt patients to immediately discontinue all medications without consulting a professional. While it is difficult for many professionals to truly know what is safe, it is even more difficult for patients. Even during pregnancy, the need to treat some illnesses outweighs the disadvantages of the medications used to treat them. This complexity is well demonstrated with bipolar disorder in pregnancy. Very few of the medications used to treat bipolar disorder have been well studied in pregnancy; however, the relapse rate for bipolar disorder for patients who discontinue mood stabilization medications may be as high as 70 percent, more than double the rate of those who stay on their medications [9, 10] – and relapse can be deadly for the mother and her fetus, especially if she becomes suicidal.

Because early pregnancy is a time of organogenesis, a review of patient medications should be conducted as early as possible, perhaps even before the initiation of formal prenatal care. We must determine which of those medications she is currently taking are safe to use, which should be discontinued, and which should be started. The obstetrical team, the addiction team, and sometimes the psychiatric care team may share this responsibility, often with the assistance of an experienced pharmacist. Online resources, such as Reprotox (https://reprotox.org), offer continually updated and concise information about the safety of medications during pregnancy.

Women with SUD are encouraged to begin prenatal care as early as possible. As soon as they become known to the team, they should be seen for initial evaluation and triage to appropriate care – not made to wait for a "new patient" opening on the provider's schedule.

## Early Prenatal Care

Patients should be educated about the benefits of prenatal care, their responsibilities, the frequency of visits, the duration of visits, and tests to be performed during pregnancy. Prenatal care begins with a thorough history of medical and obstetrical concerns, and also with a review of previous addiction and mental health care.

Knowledge of the patient's patterns of use, along with any previous treatment successes and failures, will help the care team individualize the care plan to her advantage. Is she currently using? Does she have an established relationship with an addiction provider?

Does the patient intend to carry the pregnancy? A review of the literature failed to identify studies that investigated the frequency, timing, or complications of abortion in women with SUD. Martino et al. found no association between abortion and subsequent drug use. They concluded that women who used substances were more likely to engage in behavior that led to unplanned pregnancy, but that reducing substance use would not lead to fewer abortions [11].

Pregnancy may be the patient's first experience with medical care since childhood and presents an important opportunity to introduce her to substance use treatment. Both pregnancy and addiction care represent major life events, so to face both at once can be challenging. In our experience, treatment-naive women are at increased risk of relapse through the pregnancy and postpartum.

It is important to introduce risk mitigation strategies early in the pregnancy (harm reduction). These strategies should include those intended to reduce exposure to drugs and prevention of overdose, including the prescription of naloxone. Other environmental risks, such as shared needles, should also be considered. Patients should be educated about, and assisted in avoiding, sexually transmitted infections; in this effort, clinics may consider providing condoms. Patients should be screened for a history of domestic abuse or violence. Medications the patients need in early pregnancy (prenatal vitamins with folate and anti-emetics, for example) should be determined.

Social services must be actively involved in early pregnancy to understand the resources needed for the individual patient. For patients already established and stable on MAT, care may not be much different from that of the routine prenatal patient. For many patients, needs assessment focusing on the basics must be a priority: housing, food, security, and a secure legal status. In her review of the relevant literature, Schempf questioned the degree to which poor pregnancy outcomes are related to the drug use itself versus the social, economic, and psychological factors that frequently surround drug use. She concluded that these factors would need to be addressed in order to improve pregnancy outcomes [12]. We agree that these issues must be addressed as early as possible. Furthermore, many of

these concerns need to be revisited repeatedly over the course of the pregnancy. An experienced social worker remains an invaluable member of the team throughout pregnancy and the puerperium.

The patient's initial physical examination should focus on known physical risk factors for patients with opioid use disorder (OUD). Patients who have injected medications may be at risk for hepatitis, cellulitis at injection sites, or even subacute bacterial endocarditis with associated murmurs. Laboratory evaluation should include screening for hepatitis C virus infection. Screening for sexually transmitted infections is also important at initiation of care and during the third trimester.

Prenatal genetic testing should be considered and offered, as would be done in routine prenatal care and for the usual indications. If the patient enters prenatal care early enough, she should be offered nuchal translucency, maternal serum screening, or noninvasive prenatal testing. Other options for genetic testing include chorionic villus sampling and amniocentesis. A fetal anatomical survey at the time of a second-trimester ultrasonographic examination at 18–22 weeks should also be conducted.

Smoking and OUD are both associated with increased risks of premature labor and intrauterine growth restriction (IUGR), so efforts should be made to limit or prevent both activities. Patients will often make a commitment to cut back or quit smoking before the baby is born; however, Burns et al. reported that it was harder for women with SUD to quit smoking [13]. Nurses, doctors, and other providers should utilize frequent visits in early pregnancy to stress the advantages of smoking cessation. Other centers have found that focusing on smoking cessation improves overall addiction treatment success and that this focus is more readily accepted because smoking carries a less severe stigma. Smoking cessation programs with proven success are widespread. Although the US Food and Drug Administration has not approved the use of nicotine substitutes in pregnancy, the treatment team may also consider this tool. Other medications, such as buproprion, have been studied in pregnancy and found to be successful in decreasing cravings [14]. Varenicline has not been well studied in pregnancy.

The rates of premature labor and IUGR for women with SUD are known to be higher than those for the overall population, so accurate pregnancy dating obtained in early pregnancy is vital [15–18]. In our experience, 77 percent of our patients with SUD are unable to date their pregnancy based on last menstrual period or probable date of conception, compared with 36 percent of our patients without SUD (unpublished data). Early ultrasonographic examinations are highly recommended for a number of reasons:

- To ensure viability. If a spontaneous abortion (miscarriage) is destined to occur, we believe it is preferable for our team to provide patient-centered care and emotional support, as we have found increased use or relapse to be associated with miscarriage. The pregnancy may be met with ambivalence, and miscarriage may be met with a range of emotions, including relief, grief, or self-blame. Early counseling can help the woman process these emotions and reassure her that she did not cause her miscarriage.
- To determine her due date. As stated above, this may prove very useful later in pregnancy, when accurate dating is paramount to diagnosing preterm labor or IUGR.
- If the patient plans to terminate the pregnancy, accurate dating must be known prior to referral.
- To help the patient gain a perspective on the pregnancy being real. Patients speak positively of the value of visualizing the pregnancy, and we feel that it may help to secure patient buy-in and cooperation. Some literature supports that visualization of the fetus aids in decreasing drug use and improving compliance [19, 20].

We are unaware of any untoward or negative impacts from such an ultrasonographic examination.

## Ongoing Pregnancy Care

Late or missed appointments are common among patients with SUD, so obstetric care teams need to be patient, flexible, and forgiving. Some patients may be seen only once, while others have as many as 20 visits over the course of the pregnancy. No appointment should be routine; instead, if possible, pack each encounter with social service visits, patient education, and visits with other people who can add value to her care – whether dermatology, dietary, dentistry, or other specialties – per the patient's needs. Ideally, the majority of needed services will be co-located, but if not, arranging transportation and coordinating visits can aid with compliance. Goals should be set for each visit. Consider providing healthy snacks. Ease of access to necessary services is key. Providing childcare for the woman's other children as well as transportation

improves attendance at prenatal care as well as drug treatment and should be provided if at all possible.

Throughout the pregnancy, it is important to continue to assess mental health. Zilberman et al. reported that as many as two-thirds of women with SUD also experience mental health disorders, such as depression, anxiety and panic disorders, and posttraumatic stress disorder [21]. Holbrook and Kaltenbach reported that 67.3 percent of women in an SUD program carried a diagnosis of depression, anxiety, or both [22]. Many patients are taking antidepressant, antianxiety, or antipsychotic medications, as is discussed in more detail in Chapter 4. It is critically important to make sure that the medications are safe, effective, and not causing unacceptable side effects. A number of questions concerning the patient's mental health care must be answered: Who will prescribe any related medications? How will communication be maintained to avoid lapses in treatment or abrupt termination of medications? Is the patient seeing a counselor/therapist? With proper release of information forms signed, communication between the pregnancy team and counselors should provide insight into the patient's adaptation to pregnancy and treatment for substance use disorders (SUD).

This patient population tends to have high rates of urgent care and emergency service visits [23]. We attempt to minimize these visits by anticipating when patients might seek emergency care and coach them about how to manage specific problems when the clinic is closed. Dental pain is one of the most common reasons for emergency service visits for these patients. Many have decaying or infected teeth caused by inadequate or absent dental care. They often seek emergency care to obtain antibiotics and pain medications. Providing early referrals to dentistry as well as communicating with the dental care providers on safe care of pregnant women can help prevent these emergency visits. Dental colleges, public clinics, or community dentists can be good resources to see these patients. Obstetric teams should also identify oral surgeons and prosthodontists willing to move these patients up their long wait lists to perform extractions and obtain dentures.

Drug testing during routine prenatal care is controversial. Some addiction treatment experts recommend routine testing. However, this can be problematic during pregnancy, as it increases the chance of the woman having child welfare or legal involvement without clear evidence that it improves pregnancy outcomes.

With proper consent, patients on MAT are generally recommended to undergo urine drug testing throughout pregnancy. These tests may be random or regular, depending on patient needs. Results should be shared with the addiction care team to minimize excessive screening. If urine drug testing is done, it is imperative to set a proper tone for this testing. It should be done in partnership with the patient; the goal is to demonstrate that she is remaining free of nonprescribed medications or drugs – to build a case *for* her rather than *against* her. Interpreting drug testing results can be difficult, all positive screening tests need to be sent for confirmatory testing with GC-MS if they are to be placed in the patient chart. Please see Chapters 2 and 3 for more discussion on drug testing.

## Third Trimester Care

Routine screening for glucose intolerance and anemia should be performed, as in any pregnancy. Repeat STI testing, including HIV, should be considered if risk factors persist. Obstetrical providers should follow fetal growth. Because of the increased risk of IUGR, especially with co-occurring tobacco or stimulant use, routine ultrasonographic examination at approximately 32 weeks should be considered to determine the need for increased surveillance for the rest of the pregnancy. If the infant is appropriately grown, there is no need for routine surveillance with nonstress tests unless other indications exist such as diabetes, preeclampsia, or previous stillbirth.

The care team should develop the plan for intrapartum and postpartum care management, especially pain management. Unless the prenatal provider has experience with MAT and can guarantee presence to manage intrapartum and postpartum care, a plan for pain medications in labor and management of MAT during hospitalization should be developed and placed in the patient's prenatal record (Figure 9.2). These pain management principles are discussed in Chapter 12.

Other benefits of developing a birth plan with the help of a childbirth educator familiar with the care of these women may include giving the patient an increased sense of self-control, which is important, as many have suffered trauma and mistrust the medical system, which has not always been on their side. The birth plan provides an opportunity for her to express her preferences about delivery and allows for individualized child birth education during its development. Will she breastfeed? Who will be present at the delivery?

**Labor and postpartum management for patients on methadone or buprenorphine (OMT)**

- Methadone, buprenorphine/naloxone, or buprenorphine alone, should be continued in labor and postpartum. Be aware of the patient's usual dose and schedule and try to maintain. (However, withdrawal is unlikely if the patient is receiving opioids for pain control.)
- Fentanyl may be used for analgesia, but higher and more frequent dosing may be required.
- Do not use Nubain. It is a partial narcotic antagonist which may precipitate withdrawal.
- Epidurals and nitrous oxide are OK.
- Anticipate decreased FHR variability and fewer accelerations.
- Naloxone (Narcan) may be used as a life-saving measure in the mother. Opioid withdrawal seizures may occur if used during infant resuscitation.
- A rapid drug screen should be ordered to confirm the absence of other drugs that may affect management.

**Postpartum management**

Vaginal delivery or cesarean section: continue methadone or buprenorphine. Maximize NSAIDs and other comfort measures. Hydrocodone or oxycodone-containing products may be used while on OMT. Watch the acetaminophen cumulative dose. Don't send patients home with large prescriptions. Instead, opt for quick follow-up in the clinic in 3 to 7 days.

Breastfeeding is encouraged, but not always recommended. This may depend on recent urine drug screen results.

The baby will need to stay at least 72 hours. During the time from her discharge to the baby's discharge, the patient should have her own buprenorphine or methadone to take – do not prescribe it

**Figure 9.2** A sample birth plan of management

What may she anticipate for pain control during labor or delivery? Who will provide long-term primary care for the patient (mother) after the postpartum interval? Very few patients have a primary care provider, so it may be important to introduce the patient to a follow-up clinic or provider for continued care. There is great benefit in identifying these resources with the patient before they are required.

It is also important to plan infant care. In our clinic, all patients on MAT have a visit at approximately 32 weeks with a pediatric hospitalist in our offices to discuss pediatric care, neonatal abstinence syndrome (NAS), length of stay, and so forth. Patients appreciate the enhanced education and knowing who will provide care for their baby. This visit prevents a lot of confusion and conflict and helps to set appropriate expectations regarding when the baby may go home with the mother. Identifying a clinic in your facility or a doctor in your region who regularly works with mothers with history of SUD and their babies can aid in easy and smooth referrals. Not all pediatricians are willing or able to meet the needs of these babies, and the wrong pediatrician can increase the feelings of stigma and shame these women already feel. At Gundersen Health System, a program called GunderKids was developed to provide close follow-up of babies whose mothers were considered high risk due to SUD or psychiatric diagnoses. It provides continuous support during a time of high stress for new babies and mothers, especially those mothers who might also be struggling with SUD.

The third trimester is also an important time to introduce and plan for postpartum contraception. Avoid last-minute decisions made at the time of discharge from the hospital. Long-acting reversible contraceptives (LARCs) have been strongly advised for individuals within this population [8]. If permanent sterilization is planned, provide the counseling and sign the necessary forms at least 30 days in advance of labor onset.

## The Final Month

As the pregnancy progresses into late third trimester, screening for group B streptococcus colonization should be performed. It is important to verify transportation and communication plans. It is also time for reinforcement of planning and education.

## Postpartum Care

We maintain telephone contact with our patients frequently. A follow-up visit in 2 weeks can be beneficial because screening for postpartum depression and relapse is so important in these patients. Depression and other psychiatric comorbidities may have been untreated or undertreated during pregnancy owing to fear on the part of the mother or her psychiatric provider. Now that she is no longer pregnant, we have greater latitude in treatment for depression or other medical or psychiatric disorders. A patient on MAT may have experienced a need for higher doses during the third trimester, so it may be necessary, or desirable, to begin lowering her dose to avoid over-sedation. If she has been on buprenorphine monotherapy, it may be appropriate to change her prescription to buprenorphine/naloxone. We do not encourage weaning off medication-assisted treatment in the immediate postpartum period because it is our observation that relapse risks during this stressful time are so elevated.

If third-trimester planning has been performed, postpartum care may amount to no more than

reinforcing previously made plans. If she is breastfeeding, it may be a very good time to troubleshoot any problems she may be having. The patient should have a doctor or care team to whom she may be transferred for long-term health maintenance. Contraception may be initiated, if not already begun during hospitalization. Use the trusting relationship you established with your patient during her pregnancy to reinforce the goal of continuation in therapy.

## Social Care Needs of Women with Substance Use Disorder

The elements of prenatal care for patients with SUD may be very similar to usual prenatal care. However, complicated social and legal issues may overwhelm the medical care concerns. As we noted previously, women with SUD often live chaotic lives. A broad range of resources are required in their care. Social workers serve as important connectors between the patient and the resources available. What are the patients' current needs and how likely are these to change over the course of the pregnancy? We encourage patients to take advantage of as many resources as possible. Social workers can connect them with programs available through federal, state, or local government, or through faith-based or community organizations.

One of the major challenges may be housing instability or insecurity. Patients may be homeless and living in shelters. Many are "couch-surfing" with friends or family, or potentially sharing apartments with large numbers of other people. Social workers and care coordinators are usually aware of community housing options. As patients enter treatment, they need to be encouraged to isolate themselves from drug dealers and friends with whom they have previously used drugs. This isolation can be vital to sustained recovery during the pregnancy, but it can also make the patient lonely and unable to keep working toward treatment goals. The team will need to be aware of the patient's social history and the resources and support she may call upon from a partner, family, and friends.

Many patients are transferred to doctors' offices from jail. Incarceration is not a rare phenomenon, and many patients have complicated legal problems. Some may argue that incarceration is beneficial for pregnant women because they will be safe, housed, and guaranteed to not be using. Jails and prisons are unable to provide the type of care needed by pregnant women; thus, residential treatment for substance use is far preferable. Some jails and prisons will continue MAT in pregnant women, but this is by no means universal. Many women are forced to undergo detoxification in jail, which worsens pregnancy outcomes and increases relapse risk and overdose deaths. In some states, women may be incarcerated for using drugs during pregnancy. This has not been demonstrated to be a successful strategy, and the addiction community has taken strong stands against it.

Care providers should ask patients about any past criminal charges and their current legal status. Parole officers have a lot of power over patients with criminal histories for SUD. Many will partner with health care providers to compel attendance for prenatal care. Courts may require sharing of information about patient care. In many states, drug use during pregnancy must be reported. Child Protective Services (CPS) may open files on your patients to monitor whether neonates need to be placed in foster care. We attempt to interact with CPS workers to provide our perspectives and, in many cases, advocate for our patients.

Other social and treatment goals can be addressed during the pregnancy to improve the long-term prospects of the patient's recovery. The early second trimester is an excellent time to assist the patient in setting long-term goals. For example, in our clinic, a relationship with a local community college has led to one of their counselors providing educational and vocational assessment in our office. For patients without a high school diploma, passing a General Educational Equivalent (GED) examination might be useful to future goal setting and obtaining a job. For patients who want to obtain additional training and education, grants and scholarships may be available. Pregnancy may be an excellent time to visualize and work toward a different future.

## Building Systems of Care

In this chapter, emphasis has been placed on the range and pattern of resources necessary for pregnant women with SUD. It is impossible for any one person or even several people to keep all the patients' needs met. Probably no area of health care depends more on a team of providers of different training, skills, and responsibility than addiction care. Pregnancy adds additional levels of complexity, with a mix of doctors, nurses, social workers, and other health care workers. We believe that the medical home model serves as an excellent guide for the care of these patients.

Various models of prenatal care have been described in the literature. Harm reduction models, such as those described in the previous chapter, are one example. Wright et al. described a model for harm reduction in pregnancy of substance-using women. Along with a focus on prenatal care, attention was paid to issues of transportation, child care, social services, family planning, motivational incentives, and addiction medicine. Through this model, they demonstrated a high rate of negative urine toxicology at delivery, low risks of prematurity, and high rates of retained custody [24]. Macrory and Boyd describe their program in Victoria, British Columbia, Canada, and list key components of a harm reduction program, including improved nutrition, decreased smoking, decreased alcohol and drug use, encouraging breastfeeding, encouraging physical activity, encouraging early and continuing prenatal care, and promoting social and community support [25]. In their study of the use of group prenatal care for 30 women in Lexington, Kentucky, Chavan et al. found lower incidence of neonatal intensive care unit (NICU) admission, shorter hospital stay, and lower incidence of NAS [26]. Programs such as Kaiser Permanente's Early Start have proven to be great models of coordinated care that provide excellent clinical and cost-beneficial outcomes [27].

We believe that pregnant women with SUD should be categorized as high risk, but the medical elements that make them high risk can be successfully managed by any number of health care providers who have appropriate training and experience: obstetricians, family medicine physicians, nurse practitioners, or nurse-midwives. However, what makes care for this patient population complex is not only drug use, but also the psychological, social, economic, and legal issues that they so frequently face. Thus, composition of the team may be more important than the credentials of the care providers.

The leader of the care team may not be a physician. Care coordinators, often experienced RNs, may provide the day-to-day management of these patients. The team must meet regularly, exchange ideas and plans, and always remain vigilant for problems or concerns. Trust, respect, and frequent communications are vital to keep the team performing at its highest level.

As seen in Figure 9.1, keeping the pregnant woman in the center of the care team is paramount. In our setting, the core team consists of one obstetrician, two care coordinators who divide the patient volume, two nurses, one medical assistant, and one social worker.

Redundancies are built into the structure in order to maintain the continuum of care in the absence of members of the team. Care coordinators cover each other's patients when needed, doctors are aware of social services concerns, nurses may order urine drug screens and other laboratory tests, and all of us monitor and assist each other. Team membership may vary, but communication among team members remains key.

A second ring of providers provide services in this model. This includes addictionologists, addiction counselors, psychiatrists, pediatricians, dentists, and others who have a role in supporting the care of these patients. This may include CPS case workers or members of the law enforcement and/or the judicial system. In our model, care is guided by the Pregnancy and Addiction Steering Committee, made up of the core team and representatives from each of the other groups. Strategic planning is performed at this level, and goals are set and reviewed.

We greatly value the assistance we obtain from multiple individuals in our medical center and the surrounding communities. We also see the benefits of easy and early transfer as soon as the patient reveals her pregnancy. In our setting, the addiction clinic personnel call the care coordinator, who makes an appointment for the patient to be seen in the next few days. As previously discussed, these patients should not be placed in a queue and be made to wait several weeks or a month for an appointment. The goal should be an early visit to introduce them to care and allow for successful management of patients' medications and other risks. Communication with the addiction providers must be enhanced, especially if they are independent and do not have access to the patient medical records. Release of information consents must be obtained to allow for the flow of information in this model of care coordination.

Any group of professionals should recognize their responsibilities for quality assessment and improvement. We believe it is important to establish systems of measurement, set goals, assign responsibilities, and share outcomes with other professionals, patients, and the community. Everyone benefits when patients receive the best care possible.

Our responsibility to advocate for our patients requires that we consider "Care Beyond Our Walls." We set out to build relationships in the community, such as partnering with agencies and groups to enhance housing resources that may benefit our patients. As mentioned previously, we partner with community dentists to provide dental care for our patients. Our local community college provides educational and vocational assessment for our patients. We also hope to expand our ability to provide legal consultation to our patients, as they often have high rates of noncriminal issues. Our reality is that we try to provide as much to our patients as possible with available resources. A lot of people want to help but do not know how; we can provide opportunities.

## Final Thoughts

If you do not like these patients, you will not do a good job taking care of them. Empathy and concern are hard to fake, and most patients and staff will sniff out liars and fakers very quickly. The key to survival in caring for pregnant women with SUD is building trust, communicating very, very well, and becoming a strong advocate for your patients – individually and as a group. As disheartening as it may be to see some patients return to drug use, the successes are gratifying.

## References

1. Broekhuizen F. F., Utrie J., Van Mullem C. V. Drug use or inadequate prenatal care? Adverse pregnancy outcome in an urban setting. *Am J Obstet Gynecol* 1992; 166:1747–56.

2. Berenson A. B., Wilkinson G. S., Lopez L. A. Effects of prenatal care on neonates born to drug-using women. *Subst Use Misuse* 1996; 31:1063–76.

3. El-Mohandes A., Herman A. A., Nabil El-Khorazaty M., et al. Prenatal care reduces the impact of illicit drug use on pernatal outcomes. *J Perinatol* 2003; 23:354–60.

4. Finer L. B., Henshaw S. K. Disparities in rates of unintended pregnancy in the United States, 1994 and 2001. *Perspect Sex Reprod Health* 2006; 38:90–6.

5. Mohllajee A. P., Curtis K. M., Morrow B., Marchbanks P. A. Pregnancy intention and its relationship to birth and maternal outcomes. *Obstet Gynecol* 2007; 109:678–86.

6. Heil S. H., Jones H. E., Arria A., et al. Unintended pregnancy in opioid-abusing women. *J Subst Abuse Treat* 2011; 40:199–202.

7. Santen F. J., Sofsky J., Bilic N., Lippert R. Mechanism of action of narcotics in the production of menstrual dysfunction in women. *Fertil Steril* 1975; 26:538–48.

8. Terplan M., Hand D. J., Hutchinson M., Salisbury-Afshar E., Heil S. H. Contraceptive use and method choice among women with opioid and other substance use disorders: A systematic review. *Prev Med* 2015; 80:23–41.

9. Viguera A. C., Whitfield T., Baldessarini R. J., et al. Risk of recurrence in women with bipolar disorder during pregnancy: Prospective study of mood stabilizer discontinuation. *Am J Psychiatry* 2007; 164:1817–24.

10. Newport D. J., Stowe Z. N., Viguera A. C., et al. Lamotrigine in bipolar disorder: Efficacy during pregnancy. *Bipolar Disord* 2008; 10:432–6.

11. Martino S. C., Collins R. L., Ellickson P. L., Klein D. J. Exploring the link between substance use and abortion: The roles of unconventionality and unplanned pregnancy. *Perspect Sex Reprod Health* 2006; 38:66–75.

12. Schempf A. Illicit drug use and neonatal outcomes: A critical review. *Obstet Gynecol Surv* 2007; 62:749–57.

13. Burns L., Mattick R. P., Wallace C. Smoking patterns and outcomes in a population of pregnant women with other substance use disorders. *Nicotine Tob Res* 2008; 10:969–74.

14. Cressman A. M., Pupco A., Kim E., Koren G., Bozzo P. Smoking cessation therapy during pregnancy. *Can Fam Physician* 2012; 58:525–7.

15. Center for Substance Abuse Treatment. *Medication-Assisted Treatment for Opioid Addiction During Pregnancy*. In: SAMHSA/CSAT treatment improvement protocols, editors. Rockville, MD: Substance Abuse and Mental Health Services Administration; 2008. Available at: www.ncbi.nlm.nih .gov/books/NBK64148. Accessed October 26, 2016.

16. Kaltenbach K., Berghella V., Finnegan L. Opioid dependence during pregnancy. Effects and management. *Obstet Gynecol Clin North Am*, 1998; 25(1):139–51.

17. Whiteman V. E., Salemi J. L., Mogos M. F., et al. Maternal opioid drug use during pregnancy and its impact on perinatal morbidity, mortality, and the costs of medical care in the United States. *J Pregnancy* 2014; 2014:Article ID 906723.

18. Binder T., Vavrinková B. Prospective randomised comparative study of the effect of buprenorphine, methadone and heroin on the course of pregnancy, birthweight of newborns, early postpartum adaptation and course of the neonatal abstinence syndrome (NAS) in women followed up in the outpatient department. *Neuro Endocrinol Letters* 2008; 29(1):80–6.

19. Reading A., Campbell S., Cox D. N., Sledmere C. M. Health beliefs and health care behavior in pregnancy. *Psychol Med* 1982; 12:379–83.

20. deJong-Pleij E. A. P., Ribbert L. S. M., Pistorius L. R., et al. Three-dimensional ultrasound and maternal bonding, a third trimester study and a review. *Prenat Diagn* 2013; 33:81–8.

21. Zilberman M. L., Tavares H., Blume S. B., el-Guebaly N. Substance user disorder: Sex differences and psychiatric comorbidities. *Can J Psychiatry* 2003; 48:5–13.

22. Holbrook A., Kaltenbach K. Co-occurring psychiatric symptoms in opioid-dependent women: The prevalence of antenatal and postnatal depression. *Am J Drug Alcohol Abuse* 2012; 38:575–9.

23. Coffey R. M., Houchens R., Chu B. C., et al. *Emergency Department Use for Mental and Substance Use Disorders*. Online August 23, 2010, U.S. Agency for Healthcare Research and Quality (AHRQ). Available at: www.hcup-us.ahrq.gov/reports.jsp. Accessed December 4, 2017.

24. Wright T. E., Schuetter R., Fombone E., Stephenson J., Haning W. F. Implementation and evaluation of a harm-reduction model for clinical care of substance using pregnant women. *Harm Reduct J* 2012; 9:5.

25. Macrory F., Boyd S. C. Developing primary and secondary services for drug and alcohol dependent mothers. *Semin Fetal Neonatal Med* 2007; 12:119–29.

26. Chavan N., Ashford K. B., Wiggins A., Roberts M., Critchfield A. Perinatal assistance and treatment homes for opioid use disorders in pregnancy: Impact on perinatal outcomes. *Am J Obstet Gynecol* 2017; 216;S425–6.

27. Goler N. C., Armstrong M. A., Osejo V. M., et al. Early start: A cost beneficial perinatal substance abuse program. *Obstet Gynecol* 2012; 119:102–10.

# Treatment Approaches in Women with Substance Use Disorders Who Become Pregnant

Hendrée E. Jones

## Issues Women often Face at the Time of Treatment Entry

Women who use opioids as well as other licit and illicit psychoactive substances during pregnancy often do so in the context of intricately complex social, environmental, and internal individual factors that are not usually mutually exclusive, and may be operating at varying levels and varying intensities [1]:

Social/community/external

· Gender inequality/male-focused society
· Legal involvement
· Unstable and/or poor housing conditions
· Exposure to environmental toxins and diseases
· Food insecurity

Family/home environment

· Generational drug use
· Limited parenting skills/resources
· Child abuse and neglect history
· Lack of positive/supportive relationships

Internal/biological/psychological

· Multiple drug exposures
· Violence and trauma exposure
· Lack of formal education
· Lack of job acquisition and maintenance skills
· Multiple psychiatric issues (e.g., depression, anxiety)
· Lack of nutrition
· Extreme stress

While the odds are often stacked against a pregnant woman with an opioid use disorder (OUD), each patient is unique and each patient must be viewed in the context of her own risk and protective factors to optimize her treatment and outcomes for herself and her child.

## Opioid Use in Women Who Become Pregnant

Opioid use among women who become pregnant must be seen in the context of substance use among pregnant and nonpregnant women. The most recent data from the National Survey on Drug Use and Health [2] are shown in Figure 10.1. Relative to alcohol and tobacco, that may have a more profound and lasting impact on both mother and neonate, opioid use can be seen to be relatively infrequent. Moreover, no marked difference appears between pregnant and nonpregnant women's use, as does, say, alcohol or tobacco.

The past decade has witnessed a striking increase in the use and misuse of prescription opioids by pregnant women, rising from 1.2 per 1,000 in 2000 to 5.6 per 1,000 hospital live births in 2009. The incidence of neonatal abstinence syndrome (NAS) has increased from 1.2 to 3.4 per 1,000 hospital live births during this same period [3]. More recent research has suggested that misuse of prescription analgesics (e.g., oxycodone) has risen over the period from 2009 to 2011, and suggests the possibility of a prescription opioid epidemic among pregnant women.

## Assessment of the Pregnant Woman with Opioid Use Disorder

Substance Abuse and Mental Health Services Administration (2016)[4] provides guidelines for the assessment of pregnant women with OUD. The primary aim of an assessment is to evaluate a woman's current life circumstances and her physical, psychological, and social history to determine specific treatment needs. In order to obtain as complete a picture of the patient and her past and current functioning, a thorough assessment will utilize multiple sources to obtain the necessary information, including:

• Self-report
• Clinical records

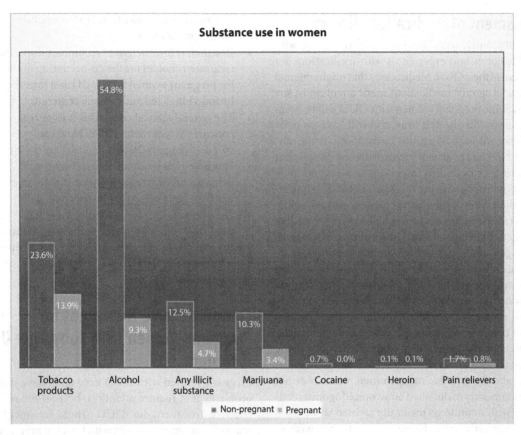

**Figure 10.1** National study of drug use and health data for women

- Structured assessment instruments
- Third-party reports
- An assessment is often the beginning of a therapeutic relationship.
- An assessment interview requires both time and sensitivity in order to elicit the necessary information from the patient. Pregnant women with opioid use disorder often have histories not only of substance use but also of trauma, physical abuse, and mental health disorders that they may be hesitant to disclose.
- Assessment should be a fluid process throughout the course of treatment – given changes in physical and psychological functioning as a result of treatment, it is critical to assess a pregnant woman periodically throughout pregnancy and the postpartum period.

The Addiction Severity Index [5] can be used in both treatment planning and assessment of treatment response, and is in wide use with pregnant patients with OUD. It gathers information in seven domains:

- Alcohol use
- Drug use
- Employment/finances
- Family/social
- Medical
- Legal
- Psychiatric

The ASI has been shown to be a valid measure with pregnant patients with OUD [6].

The prescription opioid epidemic in the USA has brought to light an economically diverse sample of pregnant women who present for treatment of OUD. They may have unique needs that are not captured by current assessment tools – and, importantly, may not be addressed by the current service models provided in comprehensive care programs. Future research is needed to determine the utility of measures such as the ASI in more affluent and diverse populations, and the potential needs for other assessment measures tailored to these groups.

## Assessment of Medication History

Pregnant women with OUD come to treatment with varied histories and experiences with medications for treatment of their OUD. Medications that might interact with opioid agonist medications merit attention in any history. Some pregnant women with OUD will be seeking treatment for the first time, and will have no prior experience with opioid agonist medications, while others may have had prior experience with one or the other medication, or both. It is important to assess not only their prior history with the medication, but also importantly, their view of the reasons for success and failure with the medication. Careful discussion with the patient can help to chart a successful choice of pharmacotherapeutic agent on the part of both patient and provider.

Other pregnant women with OUD will be seeking healthcare services for their pregnancy while already maintained on an opioid agonist. In such cases, it is likely the best course of treatment to maintain these women on their current medication, because switching medications may lead to a period of vulnerability for relapse and instability without careful patient management.

It is also the case that many women, whether or not they are currently maintained on an opioid agonist medication, wish to undergo medically assisted withdrawal ("detoxification"), often because they do not wish to expose their fetus to opioids. In these cases, it is important to discuss with these women their fears regarding opioid agonists, and in particular, how neonatal abstinence syndrome (NAS) requiring treatment does not always occur following prenatal exposure to opioid agonists, and, if it does, is a medically manageable condition.

In the final analysis, it is the patient who expresses her treatment preference. It is the role of the health care provider to ensure that the patient is fully informed as she is making her choice, and to fully engage with her regardless of her choice of treatment.

## Co-occurring Mental Health Issues

Pregnant women with OUD often have a co-occurring psychiatric disorder, and routine screening for such disorders is strongly recommended.

- Although precise estimates are lacking, it is likely that 65–73 percent of pregnant women with OUD have a co-occurring psychiatric disorder – likely a mood- or anxiety-related disorder [7, 8].
- Pregnant women with co-occurring psychiatric disorders are more likely to drop out of substance use disorder treatment, and to have poorer treatment outcomes.
- Research is insufficient to recommend specific treatment choices for the co-occurring disorder for pregnant women with OUD and thus should be individualized and patient-centered.
- The general clinical consensus is to pursue concurrent treatment of OUD and the co-occurring psychiatric disorder.
- Psychological treatments (psychotherapy, behavior therapy) may be beneficial for many patients, depending on the disorder.
- Use of psychotropic medications during pregnancy must weigh the maternal benefits of the potential reduction in the psychiatric disorder with the potential risks to the fetus of exposure to the medication.

## Comprehensive Treatment for Pregnant Women with Substance Use Disorders

Pregnant women with OUD very often have multiple problems that require attention, beyond the need for effective treatment for OUD. Thus, treatment programs for pregnant women with OUD in pregnancy in which the focus is on the mother–fetus dyad are likely to maintain these women in treatment, and minimize problems in delivery for both mother and infant. Such comprehensive programs integrate obstetric/gynecological care with substance use treatment, psychiatric care, case management services, and assistance with such services as transportation, housing, and parenting and create a recovery-oriented system of care that provides an ongoing system of support that extends beyond the formal treatment phase [9]. Figure 10.2 conceptualizes what a recovery-oriented system of care would look like for pregnant and/or parenting women. UNC Horizons, www.med.unc.edu/obgyn/Patient_ Care/unc-horizons-program is an example of such a model in action.

As seen in Figure 10.2, the main components of a recovery-oriented system of care for mothers and children are outlined below [10].

Staffing would be provided by obstetricians, psychiatrists, psychologists, social workers, family physicians, neonatologists, pediatricians, nurses, doulas, who would provide support and services throughout pregnancy and the postpartum period.

## Clinical Treatment

### Mother

- Outreach and engagement
- Detoxification
- Crisis intervention
- Counseling
- Case management
- Relapse prevention monitoring
- Pharmacotherapy
- Continuing care

### Children

- Case planning
- Residential care
- Substance use prevention
- Therapeutic child care
- Therapeutic development

### Mother and Children

- Screening
- Intake
- Assessment
- Trauma specific/informed services
- Medical and mental health care

## Clinical Support

### Mother

- Life skills
- Parenting/child development education

- Family program
- Employment support
- Link with legal and child welfare systems
- Housing supports
- Recovery community support services

### Children

- Child care
- Mental health
- Prevention services
- Recreational services

### Mother and Children

- Advocacy
- Education and remediation support

## Community Supports

### Mother and Children

- Housing
- Family strengthening services
- Child care
- Transportation
- Temporary Assistance for Needy Families (TANF) linkages
- Recovery support
- Workplace prevention
- Vocation/educational services
- Faith-based organizations

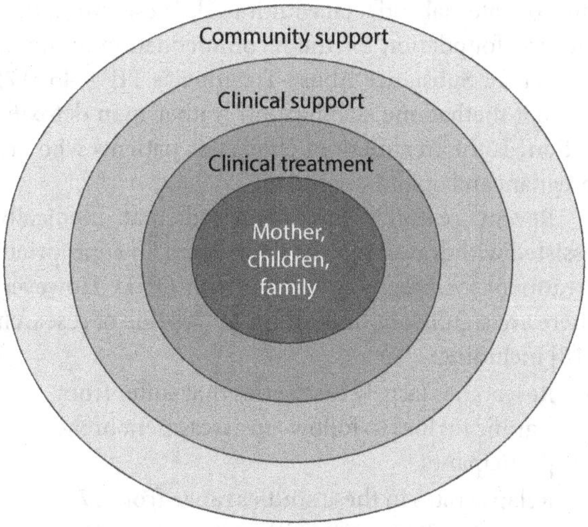

**Figure 10.2** Recovery-oriented system of care for women and children

A comprehensive care approach considers the needs of women in all aspects of program design and delivery, including location, staffing, and program development, program content, and program materials. It provides safe and comfortable environments in which women develop supportive relationships that allow them to address their recovery needs.

# Trauma-Informed Treatment

Trauma-informed treatment is not trauma-specific treatment. Trauma-specific treatment is a response to trauma experienced by the patient. In contrast, trauma-informed approach to treatment of pregnant women with OUD incorporates three key elements:

- *Realizing* the prevalence of trauma
- *Recognizing* how trauma affects all individuals involved with the program, organization, or system, including its own workforce

- *Responding* by putting this knowledge into practice

This topic is discussed in detail in Chapter 5.

# Treatment Objectives with Opioid Agonist Medication

Treatment objectives for pregnant women with OUD do not differ from treatment objectives for nonpregnant individuals. Opioid agonist medication should not be considered a cure for OUD. Methadone and buprenorphine, if used properly, can effectively suppress other opioid use. Both medications serve as critical components in a comprehensive care program for pregnant women with OUD. However, they do not change the behaviors associated with illicit opioid use. Therefore, behavioral and psychosocial interventions are needed to address the myriad of problems that pregnant women with OUD face. Moreover, such intervention can facilitate bonding between the mother and her neonate.

# Treatment Approaches to Opioid Use Disorder in Pregnant Women

Although there are certain exceptions to this general statement, there are three distinct approaches to the treatment of pregnant women with OUD:

1. medically assisted withdrawal ("detoxification")
2. opioid agonist pharmacotherapy
3. opioid antagonist therapy (not currently recommended for treatment of OUD during pregnancy)

Until recently, with the widespread licit and illicit use of opioid pain relievers (e.g., oxycodone), treatment for OUD in pregnant women had largely focused on treatment for heroin use. A critical component of such treatment has often been opioid agonist pharmacotherapy, that can include either methadone or buprenorphine [11].

# Medically Assisted Withdrawal

Medically assisted withdrawal ("detoxification") from opioids has a long and generally unsuccessful history in the treatment of OUD. Early systematic efforts to provide medically assisted withdrawal to males and nonpregnant females focused on varying short durations, often 21 days [12], although shorter (rapid and ultra-rapid) and longer [13] periods have been assessed. The general conclusion has been that medically assisted withdrawal has been a failure – although such a conclusion is now often based on the fact that some form of opioid agonist pharmacotherapy has relatively longer rates of treatment retention and less risk of overdose than medically assisted withdrawal. Slow tapering with long-acting opioids can reduce withdrawal severity; however, the majority of patients relapse to opioid use [14].

The use of medically assisted withdrawal for pregnant women with OUD has been consistently considered to be an inferior treatment choice since the initiation of opioid agonist treatment for heroin in the late 1960s in this population.

This general rejection of medication-assisted withdrawal for the treatment of OUD for pregnant women is largely based on two publications. Zuspan and colleagues [15] reported on the results of fetal monitoring of a single mid-trimester woman undergoing methadone-assisted withdrawal. Using serial amniotic fluid epinephrine and norepinephrine levels, to show a fetal-stress response, authors concluded that medication-assisted withdrawal should not be attempted without biochemical fetal monitoring. Similarly, Rementeria and Nunag [16] examined stillbirths in pregnant women addicted to heroin in a retrospective uncontrolled study. They reported a stillbirth rate of 6.4 percent for this population – there was no control or comparison condition. Also reported was $N = 1$ pregnant woman who used both heroin and methadone illicitly, and at 39 weeks, delivered a stillborn infant. She had not undergone medication-assisted withdrawal. Nonetheless, they suggested that stillbirth in pregnant women undergoing medication-assisted withdrawal may be due to oxygen insufficiency due to maternal and fetal withdrawal. These two studies laid the foundation for the recommendation found in Center for Substance Abuse Treatment's TIP # 45 [17] "... that methadone stabilization [rather than detoxification] is the treatment of choice for patients who are pregnant and opioid dependent."

Recent research has suggested that medically assisted withdrawal may be considered an appropriate treatment for pregnant women with OUD. However, there are significant limitations to this line of research [18] including:

- Research is largely case series that suffer from significant loss to follow-up assessment of the participants
- Relapse rates in these studies range from 17 percent to 96 percent, with an average of 48 percent, a likely underestimate given the loss to follow-up

- Findings do not support a reduction in the incidence of neonatal abstinence syndrome signs and symptoms (NAS) as a result of medically assisted withdrawal
- Medically assisted withdrawal is known to be associated with a higher risk of maternal relapse to opioid use, lower treatment engagement, and their attendant ancillary health risks
- There is evidence in at least two states (MD and CO) that opioid overdose is a leading cause of maternal death in the first year after delivery. Whether this increased risk of overdose is due to relapse to opioid use after a period of abstinence needs to be explored.

At present, this line of research does not support the benefits of medically assisted withdrawal in comparison to opioid agonist pharmacotherapy. Nor, has it addressed the potential longer term benefits and risks of medically assisted withdrawal for either mother or child in comparison to opioid agonist pharmacotherapy. In summary, while it may be possible to provide medically assisted withdrawal of medication to women with OUD who are pregnant, the most important questions to ask are what goals would be accomplished and at what risks to the mother, fetus, and child? Overall, the use of an acute intervention to address a chronic medical condition is not a beneficial approach for the majority of patients.

## Opioid Agonist Pharmacotherapy

There are two principal opioid agonists in wide use in the treatment of pregnant women with OUD – methadone and buprenorphine. The Food and Drug Administration's (FDA) Pregnancy and Lactation Labeling Final Rule (PLLR) went into effect on June 30, 2015. This rule discontinued the pregnancy risk letter categories (A–D and X) on prescription and biological drug labeling and now uses updated information to be more clinically meaningful to both patients and healthcare providers. The new labeling system allows better patient-specific conversations and informed decision making for pregnant women seeking medication treatment. The pregnancy letter category must be removed by June 29, 2018 [19].

Pregnant women with OUD can be effectively treated with either medication, and their use in the treatment of pregnant women with OUD should not be considered "off-label" because both medications have been approved for the treatment of OUD [20].

## Methadone

- Schedule II opioid
- Synthetically derived
- $\mu$-Opioid receptor agonist
- Also uniquely a $\delta$-opioid receptor agonist
- Antagonist at NMDA receptors
- Half-life estimated to fall in the range of 24–36 hours
- Can be provided in inpatient or outpatient settings
- Patients typically begun on methadone when they are in mild withdrawal from opioids
- Patients cannot be using benzodiazepines and alcohol before beginning methadone treatment in order to minimize chances of over-sedation
- Patients typically begin their methadone dosing under observation; first dose is small; observe for possible negative effects
- Assuming no negative reactions to initial doses of methadone, dose is systematically increased until it prevents withdrawal, cravings, and possible continued use of illicit opioids
- There is no "correct" dose; optimal dose varies greatly between patients
- Blood concentrations of patients on an equivalent dose, adjusted for body weight, have been estimated to vary between 17- and 41-fold
- Dosing does not have to be more complicated for pregnant patients

Research on the treatment of pregnant women with OUD with methadone began in 1975, following the FDA's reversal of its initial decision that pregnant women with OUD should undergo 21-day medication-assisted withdrawal, given research that suggested that there was increased risk to the fetus associated with medication-assisted withdrawal [21]. Initial recommendations were that pregnant women with OUD were to be maintained on a low dose in order to protect the fetus, and to minimize the potential for neonatal abstinence syndrome. Subsequent research suggested that low doses were ineffective in protecting pregnant women with OUD from withdrawal symptoms, and often led to illicit opioid use. Current recommendations have been to maintain a pregnant woman on a methadone dose that effectively treats her withdrawal symptoms. In line with this consensus regarding methadone dosing of pregnant women with OUD, an NIH Consensus Panel [22] declared methadone the standard of care for pregnant women with OUD.

## Buprenorphine Mono Product

- A derivative of the opioid alkaloid thebaine
- Schedule III opioid
- $\mu$-Opioid receptor partial agonist
- Primarily antagonistic actions on $\varkappa$-opioid and $\delta$-opioid receptors
- Half-life estimated to fall in the range of 24–60 hours
- Patient must already be in withdrawal or buprenorphine may precipitate withdrawal
- Patients dependent on short-acting opioids (e.g., heroin, most prescription narcotics) will not take as long to enter withdrawal as patients dependent on long-acting opioids (e.g., methadone)
- Induction typically then takes places over a 3-day period, beginning with either 2 mg or 4 mg, with a maximum dose of:
  - 8–12 mg on Day 1
  - 12–16 mg on Day 2
  - 16 mg up to 32 mg on Day 3

As a partial agonist, higher doses of buprenorphine can be given with lower risk of adverse effects (e.g., respiratory depression) than are seen with higher doses of full agonist opioids. Due to its partial-agonist effects, past a certain dose (commonly 24 mg), increasing doses of buprenorphine do not further increase the pharmacological effects of the drug but do increase its duration of withdrawal suppression and opioid blockade. Buprenorphine has a slow dissociation rate from the $\mu$-opioid receptor, which gives rise to its prolonged suppression of opioid withdrawal and blockade of exogenous opioids. This enables buprenorphine dosing to occur on a less frequent basis than full $\mu$-opioid agonists. Thus, buprenorphine can be given as infrequently as three times per week. Common adverse events experienced by pregnant women undergoing buprenorphine pharmacotherapy are constipation, sweating, nausea, headache, dizziness, hypotension, hypoventilation, and myosis. The most commonly prescribed formulation of the buprenorphine mono product in pregnancy is the sublingual tablet, available in 2 and 8 mg tablets.

## Buprenorphine+Naloxone

Both research and clinical practice with buprenorphine have almost exclusively used the buprenorphine mono product, rather than the buprenorphine+naloxone (4:1) combination product. Avoidance of the use of the buprenorphine+naloxone combination product has been based on two considerations. First, naloxone is an opioid antagonist and may precipitate withdrawal in the fetus. It appears to cross the placenta with naltrexone's presence in cord blood at delivery. However, the amount may be too small to be clinically meaningful [23]. Second, adverse effects on the fetus have been found in animal reproductive studies – although Bailey [24] argues that no known teratogenic effect has been established for naloxone use in humans when used acutely. Buprenorphine+naloxone has been increasingly used in clinical practice with pregnant women, without any seeming problems for mother or neonate based on the emerging research in this area [25, 26]. Buprenorphine+naloxone is available in both tablet and sublingual film forms, in different dosage amounts.

## Methadone *v.* Buprenorphine

Both methadone and buprenorphine are used for longer term opioid agonist pharmacotherapy, as well as for medically assisted withdrawal. Studies in non-pregnant populations suggest they are equally efficacious. They show similar adverse effects profiles, with the exception that methadone is more likely to produce sedation. However, there are two differences between the two medications. As noted above, buprenorphine is a partial $\mu$-agonist, and as such, has less potential for respiratory depression relative to methadone. However, there is the suggestion that treatment retention is more problematic with buprenorphine than methadone. As noted above, this difference may be the result of problems in buprenorphine induction.

Research with pregnant women with OUD would suggest similar conclusions regarding the relative efficacy of both medications. Both methadone and buprenorphine, in the context of comprehensive care, produce similar maternal treatment and delivery outcomes. Table 10.1 provides a comparison of methadone to buprenorphine in the treatment of pregnant women with OUD based on the available scientific evidence.

The notable difference between methadone and buprenorphine occurs in terms of neonatal response to the medication; the results below are from the MOTHER study, a randomized clinical trial comparing the prenatal exposure of methadone and buprenorphine on maternal, fetal, and neonatal outcomes [36]:

**Table 10.1** Methadone and buprenorphine: considerations for use in pregnancy

| | Methadone | Buprenorphine |
|---|---|---|
| Dosing setting | Directly observed therapy<br>Requires daily visits to a federally certified opioid treatment program; take-home medication is provided for patients meeting specific requirements | Outpatient prescription<br>Office setting – weekly or every other week dispensing/prescribing or provided in an opioid treatment program<br>*Risk of diversion may be greater* |
| First dose | 20 mg (oral) (range 15–30 mg) | 2–16 mg (sublingual) |
| During withdrawal symptoms | 5–10 mg every 3–6 hours<br>Day 2: Combined total of doses given in first 24 hours | 2 mg within 1–2 hours over time |
| Dose increase interval | Every 3 days | Every day |
| Stabilized dose | Must be individualized<br>Initial maintenance: 69 mg (range 8–160 mg)<br>At delivery: 93 mg (range 12–185 mg) [27]<br>Dividing into 2–6 doses per day the mean methadone dose engenders over 90 percent of no illicit drug use at delivery [28] | Must be individualized<br>Maintenance dose range: 4–24 mg (beyond 32 mg little increase in effect) [29] |
| Medical Complications | Maternal methadone versus buprenorphine maintenance was associated with a higher incidence of preterm labor ($P = 0.04$) and a significantly higher percentage of signs of respiratory distress in neonates at delivery ($P = 0.05$). Other medical and obstetric complications were infrequent in the total sample, as well as in both methadone and buprenorphine conditions [30] | Maternal buprenorphine versus methadone treatment was associated with a lower incidence of preterm labor ($P = 0.04$) and a significantly lower percentage of signs of respiratory distress in neonates at delivery ($P = 0.05$). Other medical and obstetric complications were infrequent in the total sample, as well as in both methadone and buprenorphine conditions [30] |
| Fetal response | Fetal cardiac measures were decreased in methadone-exposed fetuses at peak levels compared to nonmethadone exposed fetuses. Fetal Heart Rate was significantly more suppressed in the methadone plus poly drug exposure group [31]<br>Split-dosing resulted in less neurobehavioral suppression from trough to peak maternal methadone levels as compared with single-dosed fetuses [32] | Buprenorphine compared with methadone appears to result in less suppression of mean fetal heart rate, fetal heart rate reactivity, and the biophysical profile score after medication dosing and these findings provide support for the relative safety of buprenorphine when fetal indices are considered as part of the complete risk-benefit ratio [33] |
| Retention rates | Higher in treatment settings (78.1 percent) [34] | Lower in treatment settings (57.7 percent) [34] |
| Risk of overdose mortality | Higher, 4.18 per 1,000 person years in treatment [35] | Lower, 0.98 deaths per 1,000 person years in treatment [35] |
| NAS incidence | Similar (57 percent) [36] | Similar (47 percent) [36] |
| NAS treatment duration | Longer (9.9 days) [36] | Shorter (4.1 days) [36] |
| NAS and cigarette smoking | The more cigarettes smoked, the worse the NAS outcome [37] | The more cigarettes smoked, the worse the NAS outcome [37] |
| Hepatitis C | Methadone did not appear to have adverse hepatic effects in the treatment of pregnant opioid-dependent women [38] | Buprenorphine did not appear to have adverse hepatic effects in the treatment of pregnant opioid-dependent women [38] |
| Breastfeeding | Relatively safe in stabilized women [39] | Relatively safe in stabilized women [39] |
| Neurodevelopmental outcome of exposed children | No different from buprenorphine [40] | No different from methadone [40] |

- Compared with methadone-exposed neonates, buprenorphine-exposed neonates
  - Required 89 percent less morphine to treat NAS
  - Spent 43 percent less time in the hospital
  - Spent 58 percent less time in the hospital being medicated for NAS

Observational studies have shown a similar if not more robust pattern of effects between methadone and buprenorphine [41, 42].

## Agonist Medication Management during Labor, Delivery and the Postpartum Period

- Regardless of whether the pregnant woman is maintained on methadone or buprenorphine, current obstetrical guidelines recommend an epidural or spinal anesthesia for satisfactory pain management during labor and delivery.
- Agonist medications should be continued without interruption or adjustment in dose during labor and delivery [43].
- Mixed opioid agonist-antagonist medications (e.g., butorphanol, nalbuphine, pentazocine) will cause precipitated withdrawal in patients receiving opioid agonist medication and should be avoided in women receiving methadone or buprenorphine [20].
- Short-acting opioids and anti-inflammatory medications may be helpful for pain control in women receiving methadone or buprenorphine after vaginal or cesarean delivery [43, 44].

Pain management must be individualized to each mother with OUD, perhaps more so than in the case of mothers without OUD. This will be discussed in more depth in Chapter 12.

## Medication Management in the Postpartum Period

Dose adjustments must be individualized. Women during the immediate postpartum period should be closely monitored for signs of over-medication, and rarely, under-medication, and dosing adjustments made accordingly [44, 45]. Use of benzodiazepines should be closely followed given their interactions with methadone and buprenorphine to increase sedation.

Women may benefit from frequent clinical dose response assessments up to 12 weeks postpartum [45].

## Breastfeeding

Breastfeeding has many benefits for both mother and infant. This statement is equally true for new mothers with OUD. The most recent guidelines have summarized the scientific evidence shown below [39].

For methadone-stabilized mothers:

- Methadone detected in breast milk in very low levels
- Methadone concentrations in breast milk are unrelated to maternal methadone dose
- The amount of methadone ingested by the infant is low
- The amount of methadone ingested by the infant remains low even six months later
- Several studies show relationships between breastfeeding and reduced NAS severity and duration

For buprenorphine-maintained mothers:

- Buprenorphine is found in breast milk 2 hours postmaternal dosing
- Concentration of buprenorphine in breast milk is low
- Amount of buprenorphine or norbuprenorphine the infant receives via breast milk is only 1 percent
- Most recent guidelines: "the amounts of buprenorphine in human milk are small and unlikely to have negative effects on the developing infant"

The strong general conclusion is that breastfeeding should be actively encouraged for pregnant women with OUD, regardless of whether they are maintained on methadone or buprenorphine. In general:

- Hepatitis C is not a contraindication for breastfeeding (unless nipples are cracked and bleeding)
- Contraindications: HIV+, unstable recovery (this is covered in more detail in Chapter 15)

## Neonatal Abstinence Syndrome (NAS) and Its Treatment

NAS occurs not only after use of illicit opioids such as heroin, but also results from maternal use of prescription opioids and medications to treat opioid use disorder such as methadone and buprenorphine.

NAS [11] is defined by alterations in the:

- Central nervous system

  high-pitched crying, irritability

  exaggerated reflexes, tremors, and tight muscles

  sleep disturbances

- Autonomic nervous system

  sweating, fever, yawning, and sneezing

- Gastrointestinal distress

  poor feeding, vomiting, and loose stools

- Signs of respiratory distress

  nasal stuffiness and rapid breathing

The need for pharmacological treatment for NAS occurs in about 50 percent of neonates prenatally exposed to opioids. There is no single treatment protocol or medication that has proven uniformly successful. In addition to breastfeeding, other on-pharmacological strategies such as mother and child rooming together, low lights, minimal noise, skin-to-skin contact may help reduce the severity of NAS. It is important to note that NAS is *not* Fetal Alcohol Syndrome (FAS). It is treatable and to the best of current knowledge, there are no known long-term consequences from having NAS or being treated for NAS [40]. There was a significant difference between medication conditions in mean time to initiation of morphine treatment for those neonates treated for NAS, with the methadone condition requiring morphine treatment earlier than the buprenorphine condition; however, monitoring neonates for 4 days postbirth appears to be adequate to identify the vast majority of NAS events [46]. This will be covered in more detail in Chapter 14.

## Summary

Use of opioids by women must be placed in a life course perspective. Women don't chose to start using opioids when they get pregnant. The vast majority of women are using opioids and then become pregnant. Only some of those women will have an opioid use disorder. For those women with an OUD, research has shown that there are two medications that can be used as a part of a complete treatment approach, methadone and buprenorphine. For women who are already treated with methadone or buprenorphine, research and clinical experience suggests that women remain on the medication that is working for them. For

women new to OUD treatment, buprenorphine may be an optimal starting point given that the transition from buprenorphine to methadone is less complicated than the reverse. Patients will be best served through medicine when there is optimal patient-medication matching combined with individualized behavioral treatments and supports.

## References

1. Robins L. N., Mills J. L. Effects of in utero exposure to street drugs. *Am J Pub Health* 1993; 83(Suppl): 2–32.

2. Center for Behavioral Health Statistics and Quality. *2014 National Survey on Drug Use and Health: Detailed Tables*. Substance Abuse and Mental Health Services Administration, Rockville, MD, 2015.

3. Patrick S. W., Schumacher R. E., Benneyworth B. D., et al. Neonatal abstinence syndrome and associated health care expenditures: United States, 2000-2009. *JAMA* 2012 May 9; 307(18):1934–40.

4. Substance Abuse and Mental Health Services Administration. A Collaborative Approach to the Treatment of Pregnant Women with Opioid Use Disorders. HHS Publication No. (SMA) 16-4978. Rockville, MD: Substance Abuse and Mental Health Services Administration, 2016. Available at: http://store.samhsa.gov/.

5. McLellan T. A., Kuschner H., Metzger D., et al. The fifth edition of the Addiction Severity Index. *J Subst Abuse Treat* 1992; 9:199–213.

6. Jones H. E., O'Grady K. E., Malfi D., Tuten M. Methadone maintenance vs. methadone taper during pregnancy: maternal and neonatal outcomes. *Am J Addict* 2008 Sep–Oct; 17(5);372–86.

7. Benningfield M. M., Arria A. M., Kaltenbach K., et al. Co-occurring psychiatric symptoms are associated with increased psychological, social, and medical impairment in opioid dependent pregnant women. *Am J Addict* 2010; 19:416–21.

8. Fitzsimons H., Tuten M., Vaidya V., Jones H. E. Mood disorders affect drug treatment success of drug-dependent pregnant women. *J Subst Abuse Treat* 2007; 32:19–25.

9. Jansson L. M., Svikis D., Lee J., et al. Pregnancy and addiction. A comprehensive care model. *J Subst Abuse Treat* 1996 Jul–Aug; 13(4):321–9.

10. Dennis K., Young N. K., Gardner S. G. *Funding Family-Centered Treatment for Women with Substance Use Disorders*. Irvine, CA: Children and Family Futures Inc; 2008. Available at: www.samhsa.gov/sites/default/files/final_funding_paper_508v.pdf

11. Jones H. E., Finnegan L. P., Kaltenbach K. Methadone and buprenorphine for the management of opioid dependence in pregnancy. *Drugs* 2012 Apr; 72(6):747–7.

12. Del Campo E. J., John D. S., Kauffman C. C. Evaluation of the 21-day outpatient heroin detoxification. *Int J Addict* 1977 Oct; 12(7):923–35.

13. Banys P., Tusel D. J., Sees K. L., Reilly P. M., Delucchi K. L. Low (40 mg) versus high (80 mg) dose methadone in a 180-day heroin detoxification program. *J Subst Abuse Treat.* 1994 May–Jun; 11(3):225–32.

14. Amato L., Davoli M., Minozzi S., et al. Methadone at tapered doses for the management of opioid withdrawal. *Cochrane Database Syst Rev* 2013 Feb 28; (2):CD003409.

15. Zuspan F. P., Gumpel J. A., Mejia-Zelaya A., Madden J., Davis R. Fetal stress from methadone withdrawal. *Am J Obstet Gynecol.* 1975 May 1; 122(1):43–6.

16. Rementeriá J. L., Nunag N. N. Narcotic withdrawal in pregnancy: Stillbirth incidence with a case report. *Am J Obstet Gynecol.* 1973 Aug 15; 116(8):1152–6.

17. Center for Substance Abuse Treatment. Detoxification and Substance Abuse Treatment. Treatment Improvement Protocol (TIP) Series 45. DHHS Publication No. (SMA) 06-4131. Rockville, MD: Substance Abuse and Mental Health Services Administration, 2006.

18. Jones H. E., Terplan M., Meyer M. Medically assisted withdrawal (detoxification): Considering the mother-infant dyad. *J Addict Med* 2017, Mar/Apr;11(2):90–92.

19. Drugs.com. Available at: www.drugs.com/pregnancy-categories.html. Retrieved January 27, 2017.

20. Jones H. E., Deppen K., Hudak M. L., et al. Clinical care considerations for opioid-using pregnant and postpartum women: The role of obstetric providers. *Am J Obstet Gynecol* 2014 Apr; 210(4):302–10.

21. Zuspan F. P., Gumpel J. A., Mejia-Zelaya A., Madden J., Davis R. Fetal stress from methadone withdrawal. *Am J Obstet Gynecol* 1975 May 1; 122(1):43–6.

22. National Institutes of Health. Effective medical treatment of opiate addiction. *NIH Consens Statement* 1997 Nov 17–19; 15(6):1–38.

23. Wiegand S. L., Swortwood M. J., Huestis M. A., et al. Naloxone and metabolites quantification in cord blood of prenatally exposed newborns and correlations with maternal concentrations. *AJP Rep* 2016 Oct; 6(4):e385–e390.

24. Bailey B. Are there teratogenic risks associated with antidotes used in the acute management of poisoned pregnant women? *Birth Defects Res A Clin Mol Teratol.* 2003 Feb; 67(2):133–40.

25. Wiegand S. L., Stringer E. M., Stuebe A. M., et al. Buprenorphine and naloxone compared with methadone treatment in pregnancy. *Obstet Gynecol* 2015 Feb; 125(2):363–8.

26. Jumah N. A., Edwards C., Balfour-Boehm J., et al. Observational study of the safety of buprenorphine+naloxone in pregnancy in a rural and remote population. *BMJ Open* 2016 Oct 31; 6(10):e011774.

27. Albright B., de la Torre L., Skipper B., et al. Changes in methadone maintenance therapy during and after pregnancy. *J Subst Abuse Treat.* 2011 Dec; 41(4):347–53.

28. McCarthy J. J., Leamon M. H., Willits N. H., Salo R. The effect of methadone dose regimen on neonatal abstinence syndrome. *J Addict Med* 2015 Mar–Apr; 9(2):105–10.

29. Alto W. A., O'Connor A. B. Management of women treated with buprenorphine during pregnancy. *Am J Obstet Gynecol* 2011 Oct; 205(4):302–8.

30. Holbrook A. M., Baxter J. K., Jones H. E., et al. Infections and obstetric outcomes in opioid-dependent pregnant women maintained on methadone or buprenorphine. *Addiction* 2012 Nov; 107(Suppl 1):83–90.

31. Jansson L. M., Di Pietro J. A., Elko A., et al. Pregnancies exposed to methadone, methadone and other illicit substances, and poly-drugs without methadone: A comparison of fetal neurobehaviors and infant outcomes. *Drug Alcohol Depend* 2012 May 1; 122(3):213–9.

32. Jansson L. M., Dipietro J. A., Velez M., et al. Maternal methadone dosing schedule and fetal neurobehaviour. *J Matern Fetal Neonatal Med* 2009 Jan; 22(1):29–35.

33. Salisbury A. L., Coyle M. G., O'Grady K. E., et al. Fetal assessment before and after dosing with buprenorphine or methadone. *Addiction* 2012 Nov; 107(Suppl 1):36–44.

34. Gryczynski J., Mitchell S. G., Jaffe J. H. et al. Retention in methadone and buprenorphine treatment among African Americans. *J Subst Abuse Treat* 2013; 45(3):287–92.

35. Bell J. R., Butler B., Lawrance A., et al. Comparing overdose mortality associated with methadone and buprenorphine treatment. *Drug Alcohol Depend* 2009; 104(1–2):73–7.

36. Jones H. E., Kaltenbach K., Heil S., et al. Neonatal abstinence syndrome following methadone or buprenorphine exposure. *N Engl J Med* 2010 Dec; 363(24):2320–31.

37. Jones H. E., Heil S. H., Tuten M., et al. Cigarette smoking in opioid-dependent pregnant women: Neonatal and maternal outcomes. *Drug Alcohol Depend* Aug 2013; 131(3):271–7.

38. McNicholas L. F., Holbrook A. M., O'Grady K. E., et al. Effect of hepatitis C virus status on liver enzymes

in opioid-dependent pregnant women maintained on opioid-agonist medication. *Addiction* 2012 Nov; 107(Suppl 1):91–7.

39. Reece-Stremtan S., Marinelli K. A. ABM clinical protocol #21: guidelines for breastfeeding and substance use or substance use disorder, revised 2015. *Breastfeed Med* 2015 Apr; 10(3):135–41.

40. Kaltenbach K., O'Grady K. E., Heil S. H., et al. Prenatal exposure to methadone or buprenorphine: Early childhood developmental outcomes. *Drug and Alcohol* 2018 (in press).

41. Meyer M. C., Johnston A. M., Crocker A. M., Heil S. H. Methadone and buprenorphine for opioid dependence during pregnancy: A retrospective cohort study. *J Addict Med* 2015 Mar–Apr; 9(2):81–6.

42. Kakko J., Heilig M., Sarman I. Buprenorphine and methadone treatment of opiate dependence during pregnancy: Comparison of fetal growth and neonatal outcomes in two consecutive case series. *Drug Alcohol Depend* 2008 Jul 1; 96(1–2):69–78.

43. Jones H. E., O'Grady K. E., Johnson R. E., et al. Management of acute post-partum pain in patients maintained on methadone or buprenorphine during pregnancy. *Am J Drug Alcohol Abuse* 2009 Jan; 35(3):151–6.

44. Jones H. E., Johnson R. E., Milio L. Post-cesarean pain management of patients maintained on methadone or buprenorphine. *Am J Addict* 2006 May–Jun; 15(3);258–9.

45. Pace C. A., Kaminetzky L. B., Winter M., et al. Postpartum changes in methadone maintenance dose. *J Subst Abuse Treat* 2014 Sep; 47(3):229–32.

46. Gaalema D. E., Heil S. H., Badger G. J., et al. Time to initiation of treatment for neonatal abstinence syndrome in neonates exposed in utero to buprenorphine or methadone. *Drug Alcohol Depend*. 2013 Nov 1; 133(1):266–9.

## Chapter Further Reading

- www.youtube.com/watch?v=3HsmuxtsBZ8
- DRMC Neonatal Abstinence Syndrome
- http://pcmch.on.ca/LinkClick.aspx?fileticket=JTt9lpgEbN0%3D&tabid=40
- www.neoadvances.com/index.html
- www.vtoxford.org/home.aspx
- www.health.qld.gov.au/qcg/documents/g_nas5-0.pdf
- www.uvm.edu/medicine/vchip/documents/VCHIP_5NEONATAL_GUIDELINES.pdf
- http://pediatrics.aappublications.org/content/101/6/1079.full
- http://store.samhsa.gov/product/TIP-51-Substance-Abuse-Treatment-Addressing-the-Specific-Needs-of-Women/SMA13-4426
- http://store.samhsa.gov/product/Methadone-Treatment-for-Pregnant-Women/SMA09-4124

**Chapter**

**11**

# Medication Assisted Treatment for Opioid Use Disorder during Pregnancy

Lawrence Leeman and Jacquelyn Starer

Comprehensive opioid agonist treatment in combination with behavioral and prenatal care has been demonstrated to reduce the risk of obstetric complications [1]. The legal treatment of opioid dependence using opioid agonist medication in the United States is limited to two medications, buprenorphine and methadone. Opioid blocking agents such as naltrexone, and its long-acting injectable form, are also options but not yet widely used during pregnancy. Recommendations on the use of these medications will be discussed later in this chapter. Physicians and other prescribers should be cautioned that it is illegal to prescribe any other opioid agonist medications for the treatment of opioid dependence and should stay fully informed regarding current laws and regulations regarding the use of buprenorphine and methadone.

## The History of Opioid Agonist Treatment and Its Use during Pregnancy

The history behind the modern treatment of opioid use disorders, or opioid dependence as it has historically been called, dates back to the 1960s during the heroin epidemic in New York City. At the time, heroin-related mortality was the leading cause of death for young adults between the ages of 15 and 35 [2]. The original research on opioid treatment by Dole and Nyswander in the 1960s demonstrated the efficacy of methadone maintenance [3]. Pregnant women were not included in the initial research; however, treatment was eventually expanded to pregnant women [4]. By the 1970s, methadone maintenance was the recommended treatment for pregnant intravenous (IV) heroin-dependent women.

It was soon recognized, however, that maternal methadone treatment was associated with a longer and more severe neonatal abstinence syndrome (NAS) compared to maternal heroin use due to methadone's long half-life. Due to concerns regarding NAS, early regulations in 1973 required pregnant women to taper completely from her starting dose to zero milligrams of methadone within 21 days. Later in the 1970s, maintenance methadone treatment was allowed; however, the dose was recommended to be as low as possible, often 20 mg or less, in an attempt to reduce the risk of neonatal withdrawal symptoms. During this time period, it was assumed that likelihood and severity NAS were related to the methadone dose.

In the 1980s–1990s, the attitude toward methadone dosing during pregnancy changed in association with the HIV epidemic and maternal to fetal transmission of HIV among IV drug users. In the early 1990s, mother to child or perinatal rates of HIV transmission in North America and Europe were 16–25 percent [5]. Perinatal transmission was shown to be higher among women continuing to use heroin and cocaine. A retrospective review of 20 years experience of methadone treatment demonstrated that doses greater than 80 mg/day had protective value in HIV transmission [6]. The decrease in perinatal HIV transmission by treating with higher doses of methadone became a higher priority than the attempts to reduce NAS by using low doses.

In 1997, the National Institutes of Health (NIH) recommended methadone maintenance, in combination with counseling and behavioral therapy and support, as the standard of care for opioid dependence during pregnancy. The goal was and remains the treatment of maternal withdrawal symptoms through symptom-based dosing. Symptom-based dosing involves titrating the dose upwards until withdrawal symptoms, which increase the risk of relapse, are eliminated.

In 2002, buprenorphine was approved for office-based opioid treatment (OBOT) of opioid dependence and national guidelines were published in 2004 [7]. Case reports and small studies began to appear suggesting a milder NAS in infants whose mothers were treated with buprenorphine rather than methadone. This milder withdrawal syndrome is likely related to the partial agonist properties of buprenorphine compared to the full agonist properties of methadone.

In 2010, the MOTHER study compared infants whose mothers received buprenorphine to those who received methadone. The buprenorphine group of neonates required less morphine for treatment of NAS and had shorter hospital stays compared to the methadone group [8]. Numerous subsequent studies have confirmed a milder NAS with buprenorphine and no increase in adverse maternal or neonatal outcomes. The use of buprenorphine during pregnancy has become common since publication of the MOTHER study and it has become accepted as an alternative first-line treatment to methadone [9]. Patients who are prescribed buprenorphine should be counseled, however, that there is less long-term safety data available due to the limited history of use in pregnancy. Additionally, other factors in addition to the risk of NAS should be considered when selecting the optimal pharmacologic agent for an individual patient.

## Buprenorphine and Methadone Delivery Settings

Methadone maintenance treatment by law may only be prescribed and dispensed by a federally certified opioid treatment program (OTP). The Substance Abuse and Mental Health Services Administration's (SAMHSA) Division of Pharmacologic Therapies (DPT), which is part of the SAMHSA Center for Substance Abuse Treatment (CSAT), is the agency responsible to certification of OTPs. OTPs must also receive accreditation by an independent, SAMHSA-approved accrediting body to dispense opioid treatment medications and must be licensed by the state in which they operate. All OTPs must register with the Drug Enforcement Administration (DEA), through a local DEA office [10].

Buprenorphine may be prescribed in an office-based setting (office-based opioid treatment or OBOT) or in an OTP and is currently the only opioid approved for the treatment of opioid dependence in an office-based setting [5]. Specific training and a DEA waiver are required to prescribe buprenorphine. Waivers were originally limited to eligible physicians but in 2016 the Comprehensive Addiction and Recovery Act (CARA) expanded buprenorphine prescribing to include nurse practitioner or physician assistants who have also undergone specific training and received a waiver [11]. Nurse–midwives are not currently able to obtain DEA waivers.

## Women on Medication Assisted Treatment Prior to Pregnancy

Women who are using methadone or buprenorphine for MAT before they are pregnant will usually continue the same agent. If on methadone she may stay with the same outpatient treatment program or she may transfer to a program for pregnant women. As the pregnancy progresses she may need to adjust her dosing due to physiological changes of pregnancy that alter pharmacokinetics. The need for dose adjustment is most common in the latter half of pregnancy [12]. It is common to need to intermittently increase the daily dose by 5–10 mg as the pregnancy progresses, particularly in the third trimester. Not all women require dose increases during pregnancy, and dosage adjustments should be made on a clinical basis. Rapid metabolism may occur in pregnancy, especially in the third trimester, and split dosing may be indicated if the usual single daily dose does not suppress the development of withdrawal symptoms between doses. Split dosing, or dividing the daily dose into two or more doses, maintains a more stable and therapeutic serum methadone level throughout the day, which prevents withdrawal symptoms and may decrease the likelihood of NAS requiring pharmacological treatment [13].

The maternal methadone dosage does not affect the incidence and duration of neonatal abstinence syndrome based on a systematic literature review and meta-analysis [14]. Attempting to lower the methadone dose is not indicated due to concern about NAS. Women should receive appropriate dose increases to prevent opiate withdrawal and drug cravings (symptom-based dosing). Until 2001, doses above 20 mg/day [15] were deemed a contraindication to breastfeeding by the American Academy of Pediatrics; however, higher doses are no longer a contraindication based on studies demonstrating low concentrations of methadone in breast milk [16, 17].

Pregnant women on methadone may request to be transferred to buprenorphine because they have heard that neonatal abstinence syndrome occurs less frequently and is milder than for methadone exposed neonates. Pregnant women should not transition from methadone to buprenorphine solely for this reason because there is a significant risk of precipitated withdrawal, due to the long-acting property of methadone. The prolonged period of maternal withdrawal required may be accompanied by an intrauterine withdrawal syndrome with unknown fetal effects [18]. If

85

it is determined that a transition from methadone to buprenorphine is needed due to unique circumstances such as lack of methadone provider, distance to treatment or need for residential treatment which cannot accommodate methadone, then a hospital admission may be needed under the supervision of a physician experienced with this process. If she is on more than 60 mg of methadone, the transition may be difficult and the buprenorphine may not address her cravings as well as methadone, which is a risk factor for relapse [19].

Women who become pregnant while already receiving treatment with a stable dose of buprenorphine/naloxone dosage have generally been advised to continue the same buprenorphine dosage but to transition to the single-agent product. However, recent studies evaluating the use of the combination product buprenorphine with naloxone found results are similar when compared with buprenorphine alone [20, 21]. Some women may require small dose increases during the pregnancy, but this is less common than with methadone. Split dosing can also be done in pregnancy to ameliorate withdrawal symptoms.

Women can be transitioned from buprenorphine to methadone during pregnancy, if indicated, because there is no risk of precipitated withdrawal. The potential risk of unrecognized adverse long-term outcomes with buprenorphine use, which is inherent with widespread use of relatively new medications during pregnancy, should always be taken into consideration and thus a woman's request to change to methadone should be accommodated. Few women typically request transition from buprenorphine to methadone due to the convenience of buprenorphine treatment including less frequent visits along with the potential reduced severity of NAS when compared to methadone. The more likely scenario is that the buprenorphine prescriber or the obstetrician recommends transition from buprenorphine to methadone, commonly due to poor compliance with buprenorphine and the ongoing use of illicit opioids during buprenorphine treatment. The highly structured setting and observed dosing available in methadone clinics may improve compliance with MAT and abstinence.

The Food and Drug Administration approved a long-acting buprenorphine implant that provides low to moderate doses of buprenorphine for up to 6 months for treatment of opioid use disorder in patients stable on the sub-lingual form [22, 23]. The implant has not been studied in pregnant women and if a woman becomes pregnant with the implant she should be counseled regarding the lack of data on use in pregnancy However, since daily buprenorphine dosing also results in chronically elevated serum buprenorphine there is no reason to anticipate maternal or fetal harm from this delivery system. (As this book is going to press, the FDA just approved a depo formulation of buprenorphine. This will provide a greater range of options for the treatment of OUD–editor.)

## Naltrexone in Pregnancy

Naltrexone is a nonselective opioid receptor antagonist that in therapeutic doses blocks the euphoric effects of opioids and has been used to help nonpregnant patients with opioid use disorder in their effort to maintain abstinence. While the oral form demonstrates poor adherence, the more recently approved injectable long-acting form is more effective than placebo in maintaining abstinence [24]. To date, information regarding its use in pregnancy is limited to small case series and case reports, with normal birth outcomes reported [25]. However, significant concerns exist regarding unknown fetal effects, as well as risk of relapse and treatment dropout leading to return to opioid use and risk of overdose [24]. Research on naltrexone treatment during gestation poses ethical and logistic challenges but is needed to inform the use of this treatment in pregnant patients. A recent survey among pregnant women enrolled in a comprehensive substance use treatment program demonstrated a strong interest in considering antagonist treatment during pregnancy [26].

The decision whether to continue naltrexone treatment for a woman already using naltrexone prior to conception should involve a careful discussion with the patient, comparing the limited safety data versus the potential risk of relapse with treatment discontinuation. Use in pregnant women not already using naltrexone at the time of pregnancy will likely await a randomized controlled trial or prospective cohort study.

## Medically Supervised Withdrawal in Pregnancy

For pregnant women, medication-assisted therapy is the standard of care for moderate to severe opioid use disorders and is preferable to medically supervised withdrawal (MSW) because MSW is associated with high relapse rates [27], ranging from 59 percent to over 90 percent [25]. Relapse poses multiple risks, including nonmedical use of drugs, association with drug culture, accidental overdose, obstetric complications, and lack of prenatal care. However, if a woman refuses methadone or buprenorphine treatment, medically supervised withdrawal can be considered under the care of a physician experienced in perinatal addiction treatment and with the informed consent of the woman. MSW, however, often requires prolonged inpatient care and intensive outpatient treatment to be successful [28].

In some areas, access to medication-assisted treatment is limited, and efforts should be made to improve availability of local resources. Early reports raised concern that withdrawal from opioids during pregnancy could lead to fetal stress and fetal death [29, 30]. More recent studies find no clear evidence of an association between a medically supervised withdrawal and fetal death, but long-term follow-up data is lacking [28, 31, 32]. More research is needed to further assess the safety and efficacy of medically supervised withdrawal and to develop protocols. Any medically supervised withdrawal should preferably be done in the second trimester when the risks of obstetrical complications are lower. Medically supervised withdrawal should be strongly discouraged in the third trimester.

## Initiation of MAT during Pregnancy in Outpatient and Inpatient Settings

Due to the different settings in which patients may receive buprenorphine or methadone, the current delivery system often does not offer patients the ideal assessment, decision tree, and selection of medication process to individualize treatment. Although there are some OTPs that offer buprenorphine treatment in addition to methadone treatment, there are often cost considerations that prevent OTPs from doing so. The availability of buprenorphine in OTPs is currently in flux, but likely to increase. Currently, buprenorphine providers are typically clinicians in medical practice, are not licensed as OTPs, and therefore are not allowed to offer methadone treatment. Certainly, a buprenorphine prescriber can refer the patient to an OTP and OTP can refer a patient to a buprenorphine prescriber but this divided system presents obstacles and delays to a smooth transition especially when it is urgent to begin treatment, which is almost always the case. Therefore, the reality is that the current delivery system for many patients delivers a choice of medication based on which door the patient walks through.

Some programs have been developed across the country including Project Respect in Boston and the Milagro program in Albuquerque that offer hospital admission, education, counseling, prenatal care initiation, assessment, appropriate medication selection, and induction as inpatients. There are obvious advantages to this type of treatment but it has limited availability and some disadvantages as well. Some women may not be willing to spend several days in a hospital due to child-care responsibilities, work, transportation, or other issues. This type of treatment generally needs to be offered on an obstetrical unit for women with pregnancies approaching viability. To expand such programs, there is a need for more obstetricians and family medicine physicians offering maternity care to be trained and knowledgeable in MAT.

As until recently methadone was considered the "gold standard" for MAT in pregnancy, most large hospitals will have guidelines to initiate methadone for pregnant women presenting in acute withdrawal. Not all hospitals will be prepared for how to transition or refer the patient to an outpatient setting upon hospital discharge. It is critical to avoid gaps in dosing when transitioning the patient from inpatient to outpatient. It should be noted that physicians do not require special licensure to prescribe methadone or buprenorphine for hospital inpatients for the treatment of acute opioid withdrawal if they are hospitalized for another reason (e.g. pregnancy).

Patients selected for buprenorphine treatment instead of methadone treatment need to be able to self-administer the drug safely, assure safe storage, and maintain adherence with their treatment regimen. Compared with methadone clinics, the less stringent structure of buprenorphine treatment may make it inappropriate for some patients who require more intensive structure and supervision [33].

## Unique Buprenorphine Considerations

Buprenorphine has been developed as an outpatient office-based alternative to methadone, which can be used in primary care settings. For pregnant women living far from federally certified opiate treatment programs, buprenorphine can provide access to MAT through a local buprenorphine-trained provider or by traveling periodically. If a pregnant woman is to be started on buprenorphine for MAT, then it is necessary that the hospital at which she will deliver has maternity care and newborn care providers, nurses, anesthesia, pharmacy and social work that are familiar with the use of buprenorphine.

The initiation of buprenorphine treatment requires that an opioid-dependent woman go through moderate withdrawal prior to receiving her initial dose of buprenorphine. The timing can be based in part on when the patient last used heroin, fentanyl, or other opioids; however, it is important to distinguish between use of short acting agents (e.g. heroin, oxycodone, hydrocodone, fentanyl,) and long acting agents (e.g. methadone, MS Contin, OxyContin). A COWS score (Figure 11.1) of 10–12 indicates moderate withdrawal and this is appropriate timing to administer the first dose of buprenorphine which may be 2 or 4 mg sublingual. COWS scoring can vary from one institution to another so each institution should determine what score in their institution correlates with at least moderate withdrawal. Waiting for the signs and symptoms of moderate withdrawal will decrease the likelihood of precipitating withdrawal in comparison to solely using a set time since the last opiate use. It can be helpful to wait for observable pupillary dilation, which is a relatively late symptom of withdrawal and thus, if present, less likely for precipitated withdrawal to occur.

Inpatient buprenorphine induction on or near an obstetrical unit is often recommended for women who are at viability (>22 weeks estimated gestational age). Inpatient induction after fetal viability is preferable due to the theoretical risk of precipitated opioid withdrawal causing fetal stress, distress, or preterm labor. On an obstetrical setting, these adverse events can be rapidly treated. Inpatient induction also allows for better timing of the induction in relation to the progressing withdrawal symptoms. Outpatient inductions in the third trimester should probably be avoided unless in extreme proximity to an obstetrical labor and delivery unit.

Obstetrical units vary between hospitals. Community hospitals that only deliver patients at 35 weeks or above are understandably going to be reluctant to admit a preterm patient for buprenorphine initiation. Additional research is needed regarding the likelihood of preterm labor, placental abruption, fetal stress and distress, and the need for fetal monitoring during buprenorphine induction. From a practical view, we know that many pregnant women addicted to heroin are regularly experiencing more severe withdrawal than is needed to initiate buprenorphine treatment.

Prior to inpatient induction with buprenorphine women should be fully informed regarding the risks

and benefits of methadone vs buprenorphine, have a plan for ongoing buprenorphine treatment after discharge, and be informed about risks of NAS. A patient agreement may be used that includes information like a narcotics contract with the addition of information regarding effects on pregnancy and fetus, inpatient observation of infant, and options for continuing buprenorphine postpartum. Most postpartum or newborn units will require neonatal observation for 3–5 days after delivery to observe for the development of Neonatal Abstinence Syndrome (NAS) [34].

Prior to initiating buprenorphine induction at >22 weeks, there should be a documentation of a recent ultrasound to determine if there is evidence of intrauterine growth restriction. If beyond 24 weeks there should be a period of gestation-appropriate fetal monitoring such as a biophysical profile or nonstress test. If there is concern for intrauterine growth restriction, oligohydramnios or concerning antenatal fetal testing consideration should be given to initiating buprenorphine with continuous fetal monitoring on labor and delivery. If none of these conditions are present, then the induction can occur off labor and delivery without continuous monitoring such as in an antenatal unit. A urine drug screen, liver functions tests, Hepatitis C antibody and routine prenatal labs should be obtained.

Inductions may be scheduled after an outpatient consultation or may occur when a woman arrives in an obstetrical triage unit or emergency room in acute withdrawal. Ideally all pregnant women presenting in acute withdrawal requiring inpatient admission will have a choice of buprenorphine vs. methadone based on patient prior experience, polysubstance use comorbidity, and appropriateness of outpatient buprenorphine care. Women with as benzodiazepine codependence present specific challenges due to the increased risk of overdose and risk for acute benzodiazepine withdrawal. One option is admission for an observed initiation of buprenorphine or methadone with a concurrent benzodiazepine wean or phenobarbital taper (discussed in Chapter 12). Another is consultation with an addiction medicine specialist who may provide ongoing care with judicious tapering of benzodiazepines as an outpatient. Transfer to an inpatient substance abuse treatment facility once the initial opiate induction has occurred and benzodiazepine wean begun is another consideration.

The plan for administration of buprenorphine for induction can be determined based upon a patient's prior experience with buprenorphine, the severity of

# Clinical Opiate Withdrawal Scale (COWS)

## Flow-sheet for measuring symptoms for opiate withdrawals over a period of time.

For each item, write in the number that best describes the patient's signs or symptom. Rate on just the apparent relationship to opiate withdrawal. For example, if heart rate is increased because the patient was jogging just prior to assessment, the increase pulse rate would not add to the score.

| | | | | |
|---|---|---|---|---|
| Patient's Name:_____      Date: _____ Enter scores at time zero, 30min after first dose, 2 h after first dose, etc.      Times:   _____   _____   _____   _____ | | | | |
| **Resting Pulse Rate**: (record beats per minute)  *Measured after patient is sitting or lying for one minute* 0 pulse rate 80 or below 1 pulse rate 81-100 2 pulse rate 101-120 4 pulse rate greater than 120 | | | | |
| **Sweating:** *over past ½ hour not accounted for by room temperature or patient activity.* 0 no report of chills or flushing 1 subjective report of chills or flushing 2 flushed or observable moistness on face 3 beads of sweat on brow or face 4 sweat streaming off face | | | | |
| **Restlessness** *Observation during assessment* 0 able to sit still 1 reports difficulty sitting still, but is able to do so 3 frequent shifting or extraneous movements of legs/arms 5 Unable to sit still for more than a few seconds | | | | |
| **Pupil size** 0 pupils pinned or normal size for room light 1 pupils possibly larger than normal for room light 2 pupils moderately dilated 5 pupils so dilated that only the rim of the iris is visible | | | | |
| **Bone or Joint aches** *If patient was having pain previously, only the additional component attributed to opiates withdrawal is scored* 0 not present 1 mild diffuse discomfort 2 patient reports severe diffuse aching of joints/ muscles 4 patient is rubbing joints or muscles and is unable to sit still because of discomfort | | | | |
| **Runny nose or tearing** *Not accounted for by cold symptoms or allergies* 0 not present 1 nasal stuffiness or unusually moist eyes 2 nose running or tearing 4 nose constantly running or tears streaming down cheeks | | | | |

**Figure 11.1** Clinical opioid withdrawal scale (COWS) worksheet for the assessment of opioid withdrawal

their opiate use disorder and local variations regarding the availability of inpatient care. At the University of New Mexico, virtually all intravenous heroin users require 12 or 16 mg of buprenorphine to manage withdrawal symptoms. A protocol to quickly eliminate withdrawal includes an initial dose of 4 mg based on COWS score consistent with moderate withdrawal which is repeated 30–60 minutes later if withdrawal was not precipitated by the first dose. A third 4 mg dose is then given 2 hours later. An additional dose is given if the COWS score and examination are consistent with ongoing withdrawal. At times, escalation to 20 or 24 mg in the first 24 hours is required which is higher than recommended during the first day of an outpatient buprenorphine induction. The finding that the trajectory of rising opiate withdrawal scores was higher in the Mother study suggests that a more rapid induction may potentially decrease the likelihood of an unsuccessful buprenorphine induction [35]. Medications to treat withdrawal symptoms may include acetaminophen, Phenergan, and Lomotil (Diphenoxylate/Atropine).

After buprenorphine inpatient induction the patient can be discharged when stable if she has a safe social situation and appropriate housing. If the first follow-up appointment is going to be delayed, then she may be observed for a longer period. One approach is to start buprenorphine inductions in the morning, to achieve an adequate buprenorphine dose to eliminate acute withdrawal within four hours and then, if she remains inpatient, she will receive the next morning dose equivalent to the total first day dose.

Once acute withdrawal has been treated and the patient observed for a minimum of 8–12 hours, she may be discharged home to follow up with outpatient care for MAT. Due to the chaotic life of many intravenous heroin users, a few additional days for stabilization, addressing medical or psychiatric comorbidities, and ensuring safe stable housing is often needed.

Women who will be transferred to a jail or prison after started on MAT represent a potentially challenging situation. As it is common for incarcerated women to have a limited ability to access care for dose increases it is preferable to keep them inpatient until stable daily dose is identified. Prisons vary widely regarding their ability and willingness to maintain pregnant women on MAT and some have a policy requiring all incarcerated patients to go through withdrawal/detoxification without access to methadone or buprenorphine using only medications to treat symptoms [28]. The buprenorphine implant may be considered in this situation.

These policies are unethical and all efforts should be made to change these laws and policies through physician advocacy.

## Unique Methadone Considerations

Methadone is a pure agonist and there is not a need for the patient to be in moderate withdrawal to avoid precipitated withdrawal. Initiation as an outpatient is considered appropriate throughout pregnancy. Methadone may be started at 20–30 mg/day. If withdrawal continues despite this initial dose, then an additional 5–10 mg may be given each day as a rescue dose and added to the next day's morning dose if in an inpatient setting. As methadone has a long half-life a steady state is not achieved for 5–7 days. It is essential that the dose not be increased too rapidly since the serum level will continue to increase for several days after the increase, which may lead to risks associated with overmedication and overdose [36]. By the 5th day of methadone use the dose should not be greater than 50–60 mg and additional increases of 5–10 mg can then occur as needed at 3–4 day intervals. Although the time of day of initial treatment may be any hour of the day based on withdrawal symptoms and time of admission the goal is to transition to a morning dose for outpatient treatment. Women who are started as outpatients frequently "supplement" their daily methadone dose with continued use of heroin or prescription opioids until the daily dose is high enough to relieve withdrawal symptoms and cravings.

Methadone can prolong the cardiac QTc interval which can lead to the potentially fatal torsades de pointes ventricular arrhythmia. Methadone interacts with several other drugs which may affect methadone levels or directly increase the cardiac QTc interval including some antiretroviral HIV medications, fluconazole and fluoroquinolones [37]. A baseline EKG should be done prior to initiating methadone treatment. If the QTc interval is >500 ms then use of methadone is not recommended [38]. If the QTc is between 450 and 500 ms then methadone can be used, however a repeat EKG should be done after 2–3 weeks of use [38]. All pregnant women should have a repeat EKG when the dose reaches 100 mg/day [38].

## Summary

This chapter is intended to provide adequate information to understand and implement optimal management of the various treatment modalities involved in the management of opioid use disorders during pregnancy with MAT. Pregnant women with OUDs will require a treatment team to coordinate optimal care. Obstetricians and other prenatal care providers may play a role in prescribing opioid agonist medication or they may work in conjunction with addiction medicine specialists, primary care physicians offering buprenorphine treatment, and OTPs. OUD in pregnancy used to be primarily urban-based heroin use and there were minimal geographic barriers to methadone-based MAT. In the current opiate epidemic, the widespread misuse of prescription opioids has spread OUD in pregnancy to many rural and smaller communities without access to methadone treatment. The increasing use of buprenorphine as part of MAT in pregnancy has increased access to treatment; however, there is a large unmet need for care of pregnant women with OUD and their infants who commonly require prolonged treatment for neonatal abstinence syndrome.

# References

1. Jones H. E., Martin P. R., Heil S. H., et al. Treatment of opioid-dependent pregnant women: clinical and research issues. *Journal of Substance Abuse Treatment*. Oct 2008;35(3):245–59.

2. Joseph H., Dole V. P. Methadone patients on probation and parole. *Federal probation*. Jun 1970;34:42–8.

3. Dole V. P., Nyswander M. A medical treatment for diacetylmorphine (heroin) addiction. A clinical trial with methadone hydrochloride. *JAMA*. Aug 23 1965;193:646–50.

4. Blinick G., Jerez E., Wallach R. C. Methadone maintenance, pregnancy, and progeny. *JAMA*. Jul 30 1973;225(5):477–9.

5. Treatment CfSA. *Medication-Assisted Treatment for Opioid Addiction in Opioid Treatment Programs*. Treatment Improvement Protocol (TIP) Series, No. 43. Center for Substance Abuse Treatment. Rockville, MD: Substance Abuse and Mental Health Services Administration (US); 2005.

6. Hartel D. M., Schoenbaum E. E. Methadone Treatment Protects against HIV Infection: Two Decades of Experience in the Bronx, New York City. *Public Health Reports (Washington, D.C.: 1974)*. Jun 1998;113(Suppl 1):107–15.

7. Treatment CfSA. *Clinical Guidelines for the Use of Buprenorphine in the Treatment of Opioid Addiction*. Treatment Improvement Protocol (TIP) Series, No. 40. Center for Substance Abuse Treatment. Rockville, MD: Substance Abuse and Mental Health Services Administration (US); 2004.

8. Jones H. E., Kaltenbach K., Heil S. H., et al. Neonatal abstinence syndrome after methadone or buprenorphine exposure. *The New England Journal of Medicine*. Dec 9 2010;363(24):2320–31.

9. ACOG Committee. Opinion No. 524: Opioid abuse, dependence, and addiction in pregnancy. *Obstetrics and Gynecology*. May 2012;119(5):1070–6.

10. SAMHSA. *Certification of Opioid Treatment Programs (OTPs)*. 2015; www.samhsa.gov/medication-assisted-treatment/opioid-treatment-programs. Accessed January 6, 2017.

11. American Society of Addiction Medicine. *Nurse Practitioners and Physician Assistants Prescribing Buprenorphine*. www.asam.org/quality-practice/practice-resources/nurse-practitioners-and-physician-assistants-prescribing-buprenorphine. Accessed February 25, 2017.

12. Pond S. M., Kreek M. J., Tong T. G., Raghunath J., Benowitz N. L. Altered methadone pharmacokinetics in methadone-maintained pregnant women. *The Journal of Pharmacology and Experimental Therapeutics*. Apr 1985;233(1):1–6.

13. McCarthy J. J., Leamon M. H., Willits N. H., Salo R. The effect of methadone dose regimen on neonatal abstinence syndrome. *Journal of Addiction Medicine*. Mar–Apr 2015;9(2):105–10.

14. Cleary B. J., Donnelly J., Strawbridge J., et al. Methadone dose and neonatal abstinence syndrome – systematic review and meta-analysis. *Addiction (Abingdon, England)*. Dec 2010;105(12):2071–84.

15. American Academy of Pediatrics Committee on Drugs: The transfer of drugs and other chemicals into human milk. *Pediatrics*. Jan 1994;93(1):137–50.

16. Jansson L. M., Choo R., Velez M. L., et al. Methadone maintenance and breastfeeding in the neonatal period. *Pediatrics*. Jan 2008;121(1):106–14.

17. American Academy of Pediatrics Committee on Drugs. Transfer of drugs and other chemicals into human milk. *Pediatrics*. Sep 2001;108(3):776–89.

18. McCarthy J. J. Intrauterine abstinence syndrome (IAS) during buprenorphine inductions and methadone tapers: can we assure the safety of the fetus? *The Journal of Maternal-Fetal & Neonatal Medicine: The Official Journal of the European Association of Perinatal Medicine, the Federation of Asia and Oceania Perinatal Societies, the International Society of Perinatal Obstet*. Feb 2012;25(2):109–12.

19. Mannelli P., Peindl K. S., Lee T., Bhatia K. S., Wu L. T. Buprenorphine-mediated transition from opioid agonist to antagonist treatment: state of the art and new perspectives. *Current Drug Abuse Reviews*. Mar 2012;5(1):52–63.

20. Debelak K., Morrone W. R., O'Grady K. E., Jones H. E. Buprenorphine + naloxone in the treatment of opioid dependence during pregnancy–initial patient care and outcome data. *The American Journal on Addictions.* May–Jun 2013;22(3):252–4.

21. Wiegand S. L., Stringer E. M., Stuebe A. M., et al. Buprenorphine and naloxone compared with methadone treatment in pregnancy. *Obstetrics and Gynecology.* Feb 2015;125(2):363–8.

22. Rosenthal R. N., Lofwall M. R., Kim S., et al. Effect of buprenorphine implants on illicit opioid use among abstinent adults with opioid dependence treated with sublingual buprenorphine: a randomized clinical trial. *JAMA.* Jul 19 2016;316(3):282–90.

23. Sigmon S. C., Bigelow G. E. Food and Drug Administration approval of sustained-release buprenorphine for treatment of opioid dependence: realizing its potential. *Addiction (Abingdon, England).* Mar 2017;112(3):386–7.

24. Jones H. E., Chisolm M. S., Jansson L. M., Terplan M. Naltrexone in the treatment of opioid-dependent pregnant women: the case for a considered and measured approach to research. *Addiction (Abingdon, England).* Feb 2013;108(2):233–47.

25. Saia K. A., Schiff D., Wachman E. M., et al. Caring for pregnant women with opioid use disorder in the USA: expanding and improving treatment. *Current Obstetrics and Gynecology Reports.* 2016;5:257–63.

26. Jones H. E. Acceptance of naltrexone by pregnant women enrolled in comprehensive drug addiction treatment: an initial survey. *The American Journal on Addictions.* May–Jun 2012;21(3):199–201.

27. Jones H. E., O'Grady K. E., Malfi D., Tuten M. Methadone maintenance vs. methadone taper during pregnancy: maternal and neonatal outcomes. *The American Journal on Addictions.* Sep–Oct 2008;17(5):372–86.

28. Bell J., Towers C. V., Hennessy M. D., et al. Detoxification from opiate drugs during pregnancy. *American Journal of Obstetrics and Gynecology.* Sep 2016;215(3):374 e371–76.

29. Rementeria J. L., Nunag N. N. Narcotic withdrawal in pregnancy: stillbirth incidence with a case report. *American Journal of Obstetrics and Gynecology.* Aug 15 1973;116(8):1152–6.

30. Zuspan F. P., Gumpel J. A., Mejia-Zelaya A., Madden J., Davis R. Fetal stress from methadone withdrawal. *American Journal of Obstetrics and Gynecology.* May 1 1975;122(1):43–6.

31. Luty J., Nikolaou V., Bearn J. Is opiate detoxification unsafe in pregnancy? *Journal of Substance Abuse Treatment.* Jun 2003;24(4):363–7.

32. Welle-Strand G. K., Skurtveit S., Tanum L., et al. Tapering from methadone or buprenorphine during pregnancy: maternal and neonatal outcomes in Norway 1996–2009. *European Addiction Research.* 2015;21(5):253–61.

33. Alto W. A., O'Connor A. B. Management of women treated with buprenorphine during pregnancy. *American Journal of Obstetrics and Gynecology.* Oct 2011;205(4):302–8.

34. Hudak M. L., Tan R. C. Neonatal drug withdrawal. *Pediatrics.* Feb 2012;129(2):e540–60.

35. Holbrook A. M., Jones H. E., Heil S. H., et al. Induction of pregnant women onto opioid-agonist maintenance medication: an analysis of withdrawal symptoms and study retention. *Drug and Alcohol Dependence.* Sep 1 2013;132(1–2):329–34.

36. Srivastava A., Kahan M. Methadone induction doses: are our current practices safe? *Journal of Addictive Diseases.* 2006;25(3):5–13.

37. McCance-Katz E. F., Sullivan L. E., Nallani S. Drug interactions of clinical importance among the opioids, methadone and buprenorphine, and other frequently prescribed medications: a review. *The American Journal on Addictions.* Jan–Feb 2010;19(1):4–16.

38. Chou R., Cruciani R. A., Fiellin D. A., et al. Methadone safety: a clinical practice guideline from the American Pain Society and College on Problems of Drug Dependence, in collaboration with the Heart Rhythm Society. *The Journal of Pain: Official Journal of the American Pain Society.* Apr 2014;15(4):321–37.

# Chapter 2

# Labor and Delivery Management in Women with Substance Use Disorder

Marjorie Meyer and Tricia E. Wright

Labor and delivery is a stressful place for patients and staff. As a combination emergency department, intensive care unit, operating room, and birthing center, both patients and staff bring a heterogeneous mix of expectations and clinical skills to the bedside. For women with substance use disorders, the additional stresses of guilt and concerns of judgment by caregivers, as well as the effects of past trauma, heighten the anxiety. In this chapter, we will review the labor and delivery management of women with substance use disorders, with an emphasis on opioid-dependent patients.

## Admission in the Setting of Acute Intoxication/Withdrawal

Those caring for women with substance use disorders have a few special considerations when they are admitted to labor and delivery. Those include treating acute intoxication or withdrawal, managing pain appropriately, providing trauma-informed care, and addressing infectious disease concerns. Infectious disease screens and liver and renal function evaluation should be repeated if ongoing illicit use is suspected (especially HIV, hepatitis B, and syphilis since intrapartum and immediate newborn management may be altered). Given that most women with opioid use disorders use multiple substances, special considerations must be given to those substances whose use and withdrawal pose an immediate risk of harm to the pregnant woman and fetus.

**Alcohol:** Women who have been misusing alcohol during pregnancy have specific risks when admitted to labor and delivery. Women presenting with acute intoxication may be agitated and combative. Serum glucose should be assessed at admission as hypoglycemia may exacerbate behavior issues. Women with AUD are frequently dehydrated and benefit from IV hydration. Thiamine (100 mg) should be added to IV fluids to prevent Wernicke's encephalopathy [1]. For control of agitation that interferes with patient care, short

acting benzodiazepines (midazolam) may be indicated to allow initial evaluation and fetal assessment. Women presenting with chronic alcohol use during pregnancy are at risk for withdrawal during the course of hospitalization even in the absence of obvious intoxication. Serial evaluation for alcohol withdrawal can be performed with the CIWA-Ar scale (Figure 12.1), with intermittent doses of a long acting benzodiazepine (chlordiazepoxide (Librium®) 25–50 mg, diazepam (Valium®) 5–10 mg, or lorazepam (Ativan®) 1–2 mg) for scores greater than 8 [2, 3]. Mild withdrawal can occur by 6 hours of abstinence; hallucinosis after 12–24 hours of abstinence; withdrawal seizures after 12–48 hours of abstinence; and delirium tremens (hallucinations, disorientation, tachycardia, hypertension, hyperthermia, agitation, diaphoresis) after 48–96 hours of abstinence. Delirium tremens is most common in older individuals (age 40–50) with long-standing chronic alcohol use. Common obstetric complications such as preeclampsia or hyperthyroidism that can mimic alcohol withdrawal should be carefully considered in the differential diagnosis. Obstetric providers should work closely with other medical providers (emergency room colleagues would be helpful if no addiction specialist is available) to diagnose and treat alcohol withdrawal and titrate medications. Benzodiazepines are the mainstay for the prevention and treatment of alcohol withdrawal and should be administered as indicated. Pediatricians should be made aware of both alcohol exposure and benzodiazepine treatment if required, with availability for respiratory support of the neonate if high doses of benzodiazepines are needed.

**Benzodiazepine misuse:** Benzodiazepines are commonly misused with other illicit substances, complicating specific identification and treatment. Oral benzodiazepine misuse alone does not usually cause severe respiratory depression; patients present with depressed mental status but no other findings, the "coma with normal vital signs." Standard supportive care is indicated. Many benzodiazepines will not

# The Clinical Institute Withdrawal Assessment for Alcohol—Revised

### Addiction Research Foundation Clinical Institute Withdrawal Assessment for Alcohol (CIWA-Ar)

Patient _____  Date |—|—|—|  Time ____:____
                                                         Y  m  d   (24-hour clock, midnight=00:00)

Pulse or heart rate, taken for one minute: _____          Blood pressure: _____ / _____

**NAUSEA AND VOMITING—Ask "Do you feel sick to your stomach? Have you vomited?" Observation.**
0 no nausea and no vomiting
1 mild nausea with no vomiting
2
3
4 intermittent nausea with dry heaves
5
6
7 constant nausea, frequent dry heaves and vomiting

**TREMOR—Arms extended and fingers spread apart. Observation.**
0 no tremor
1 not visible, but can be felt fingertip to fingertip
2
3
4 moderate, with patient's arm extended
5
6
7 severe, even with arms not extended

**PAROXYSMAL SWEATS—Observation.**
0 no sweat visible
1 barely perceptible sweating, palms moist
2
3
4 beads of sweat obvious on forehead
5
6
7 drenching sweats

**ANXIETY—Ask "Do you feel nervous?" Observation.**
0 no anxiety, at ease
1 mildly anxious
2
3
4 moderately anxious, or guarded, so anxiety is inferred
5
6
7 equivalent to acute panic states as seen in severe delirium or acute schizophrenic reactions

**AGITATION—Observation.**
0 normal scarcity
1 somewhat more than normal activity
2
3
4 moderately fidgety and restless
5
6
7 paces back and forth during most of the interview, or constantly thrashes about

**TACTILE DISTURBANCES—Ask "Have you any itching, pins and needles sensations, any burning, any numbness, or do you feel bugs crawling on or under your skin?" Observation.**
0 none
1 very mild itching, pins and needles, burning or numbness
2 mild itching, pins and needles, burning or numbness
3 moderate itching, pins and needles, burning or numbness
4 moderately severe hallucinations
5 severe hallucinations
6 extremely severe hallucinations
7 continuous hallucinations

**AUDITORY DISTURBANCES—Ask "Are you more aware of sounds around you? Are they harsh? Do they frighten you? Are you hearing anything that is disturbing to you? Are you hearing things you know are not there?" Observation.**
0 not present
1 very mild harshness or ability to frighten
2 mild harshness or ability to frighten
3 moderate harshness or ability to frighten
4 moderately severe hallucinations
5 severe hallucinations
6 extremely severe hallucinations
7 continuous hallucinations

**VISUAL DISTURBANCES—Ask "Does the light appear to be too bright? Is its color different? Does it hurt your eyes? Are you seeing anything that is disturbing to you? Are you seeing things you know are not there?" Observation.**
0 not present
1 very mild sensitivity
2 mild sensitivity
3 moderate sensitivity
4 moderately severe hallucinations
5 severe hallucinations
6 extremely severe hallucinations
7 continuous hallucinations

**HEADACHE, FULLNESS IN HEAD—Ask "Does your head feel different? Does it feel like there is a band around your head?" Do not rate for dizziness or lightheadedness. Otherwise, rate severity.**
0 not present
1 very mild
2 mild
3 moderate
4 moderately severe
5 severe
6 very severe
7 extremely severe

**ORIENTATION AND CLOUDING OF SENSORIUM— Ask "What day is this? Where are you? Who am I?"**
0 oriented and can do serial additions
1 cannot do serial additions or is uncertain about date
2 disoriented for date by no more than 2 calendar days
3 disoriented for date by more than 2 calendar days
4 disoriented for place and/or person

Total CIWA-Ar Score____
Rater's Initials____
Maximum Possible Score 67

This scale is not copyrighted and may be used freely.

**Figure 12.1** The Clinical Institute Withdrawal Assessment for Alcohol-Revised (CIWA-Ar)

be identified by routine urine drug screen (clonazepam, lorazepam), thus the diagnosis requires a high level of suspicion, and specific drug screens ordered. Reversal of benzodiazepine effect with flumazenil should be avoided: flumazenil does not reverse respiratory depression and acute reversal can precipitate seizures in chronic benzodiazepine users. The risk/benefit does NOT favor reversal with flumazenil [4]. Benzodiazepine withdrawal can occur after chronic, long-term use; symptoms include seizures, tremors, perceptual disturbance, and psychosis.

There are three options for treatment of chronic benzodiazepine use.

1. Treatment with long-acting benzodiazepines (chlordiazepoxide 25–50 mg or lorazepam 5–10 mg) during the hospitalization with referral to outpatient treatment for taper postpartum.
2. Taper with long-acting benzodiazepines (chlordiazepoxide 25–50 mg or lorazepam 5–10 mg) during the hospital course based on symptoms and CIWA-B scores.
3. Taper with phenobarbital during the hospital course. This taper was first reported by Kawasaki et al. [5] and has been used often in our center with good results. This taper has the advantage of not requiring use of specialized scoring systems (such as CIWA-B), which require nursing training.

The latter two options are useful for women who will be entering residential treatment centers without capability for benzodiazepine taper upon release.

**Cocaine/methamphetamine use:** Both cocaine and methamphetamine intoxication are characterized by profound sympathetic overload: hypertension, cardiovascular derangements including tachycardia and ischemia, and cardiovascular collapse [6]. Acute intoxication is treated with supportive measures but other diseases such as preeclampsia and hyperthyroidism should be excluded. It is critical to differentiate stimulant intoxication from other etiologies of hypertension (i.e., preeclampsia, hyperthyroidism); neither beta blockers nor labetalol should be used for the treatment of hypertension related to cocaine or amphetamine intoxication. Beta blockade in the setting of cocaine intoxication can cause unopposed alpha adrenergic stimulation, coronary vasoconstriction, or end organ ischemia. In the absence of acute hypertensive crisis, first line therapy should be benzodiazepines (diazepam 10 mg then 5–10 mg q 3–5 minutes); this approach reduces the central catecholamine release rather than

blocking peripheral action. If additional medication for hypertension is required, the alpha antagonist phentolamine is the treatment of choice, with nitroglycerine added for cocaine-associated chest pain. Any antihypertensive therapy should be carefully titrated, as the effects of amphetamines or cocaine can be short lived and self-limiting, and overtreatment and hypotension may occur suddenly. Anesthetic management in the setting of cocaine intoxication is complicated: succinylcholine and cocaine are both metabolized by plasma cholinesterase, so the effects of both medications may be prolonged; anesthesia induction in the setting of acute hypertension can be dangerous; effects of inhaled anesthetic agents can be modified by amphetamines. Given the high rate of pregnancy complications (abruption, nonreassuring fetal assessment) that might lead to emergent cesarean delivery, early consultation with anesthesiology should be requested. It is always important to note that correction of maternal cardiovascular derangements can often improve fetal status and allow prolongation of pregnancy.

**Opioid intoxication/withdrawal:** Treatment for opioid intoxication is supportive, including respiratory support as needed. It is of note that pulse oximetry can be used to assess oxygenation but not ventilation. End tidal $CO_2$ or arterial blood gas measurements should be used to monitor ventilation if respiratory depression is observed. Reversal with naloxone should be used only to reverse respiratory depression, not to normalize mental status. If withdrawal is inadvertently precipitated by naloxone, treatment should be supportive as naloxone has a short half-life. Women presenting with acute opioid withdrawal can be stabilized with a short acting full opioid agonist (such as fentanyl 50–100 mcg) until a definitive treatment plan can be developed or with methadone 10 mg. It is of note that if buprenorphine is likely to be the long-term medication of choice, short-term stabilization with short acting opioids rather than the longer acting methadone may be preferable due to ease of transition to buprenorphine.

**Other substances:** There are few data regarding various synthetic agents, bath salts, inhalation agents, etc. Most of these substances require supportive care and are often used with other more commonly misused medications. Pregnancy specific data are limited.

**Approach to the patient with unknown intoxicants:** Unfortunately, most illicit drugs do not travel alone, so the guidelines outlined above may require modification. Talking with addiction medicine or emergency room colleagues can give a sense of which drugs are present in a given community. Clinicians can also get a sense of the most predominant drug at presentation based on physical exam. Patients presenting with agitation, paranoia, and hallucinations with tachycardia, hypertension, and tachypnea are under the predominant effect of sympathomimetics (methamphetamines, cocaine), anticholinergics (belladonna alkyloids), or hallucinogens (PCP, LSD, MDMA). The presence of nystagmus is more suggestive of hallucinogens; urinary retention is more common with anticholinergics, and tremors, seizures, and hyperreflexia more characteristic of sympathomimetics. Patients presenting with depressed mental status often have bradycardia, hypotension, and bradypnea. Serotonin syndrome more often has mydriasis, as opposed to opioids or sedative/hypnotics which may have miosis. Rapid lab evaluation can help identify alcohol levels and urine drug screen may identify opioids, which can assist with the differential. Supportive care will be similar for all.

Substance use (and cigarette smoking) is associated with fetal growth restriction; assessment of fetal weight clinically or with ultrasound will facilitate planning for monitoring, delivery, and newborn care. Admission urine drug screen may be of assistance for all patients with substance use disorder to assist the pediatric management. All urine drug testing must be done with the patient's consent and explanation as to what the results will be used for.

## Fetal Assessment in the Setting of Intoxication/Withdrawal

Fetal monitoring is influenced by both uteroplacental perfusion and the direct effect of the intoxicant. As with many other maternal illnesses, correction of maternal physiology can improve fetal status. When feasible, optimization of maternal status should be performed before delivery for nonreassuring fetal status due to substance intoxication.

Uterine perfusion can be compromised by acute maternal hypertension or vasospasm, which can occur with stimulant use or acute opioid withdrawal. Treatment should be directed as noted above, with benzodiazepines to decrease sympathetic output with stimulant use or opioid agonists to reverse opioid withdrawal. Unfortunately, both benzodiazepines and opioids can then lead to decreased fetal heart rate variability and decreased fetal movement; careful titration

can minimize these effects. Similarly, fetal activity on ultrasound may be reduced so additional testing such as biophysical profile assessment should be interpreted with caution [7]. Both alcohol and opioid intoxication have been associated with reduced fetal heart rate variability and late decelerations which improve with resolution of intoxication. There are no data to guide the difficult decision of conservative management versus delivery in the setting of non-reassuring fetal assessment. This decision will be a complicated assessment of gestational age, fetal status and ability to improve maternal physiology to achieve fetal recovery. Assessment of fetal acid base status by umbilical cord blood gas analysis at the time of delivery will assist the pediatricians in the evaluation of the infant.

## Admission (Routine) and Intrapartum Management

Most women with substance use disorder will not present with acute intoxication or withdrawal, but rather in labor or for planned delivery. Infectious disease screens and liver and renal function evaluation should be repeated if ongoing illicit use or misuse is suspected. Women that admit to chronic alcohol or untreated chronic opioid use should be followed for withdrawal symptoms and treated accordingly. Urine drug screen at admission should be performed to assist the pediatricians in the evaluation of the neonate with permission of the mother and disclosure as to how the results will be used. If the woman refuses testing, careful explanation should be given as to its importance in a nonjudgmental manner. Women have valid fears of drug screening: positive tests have been used for prosecution and loss of custody. Clinicians should advocate for treatment as opposed to punishment in their communities. Urine drug screens are limited in the detection of illicit drug use: the assays have limited detection of commonly misused opioids (fentanyl, oxycodone) and some substances have very short excretion windows (i.e. cocaine). These limitations can be overcome with a careful history and explanation regarding the importance of disclosure for optimal neonatal care. For the rest of intrapartum and postpartum care, women with alcohol, cocaine, or other substance use is unchanged from the standard of care.

Women with opioid use disorder (OUD), however, have specific considerations which are discussed in detail below. Women receiving medication assisted therapy (MAT) should continue medication as scheduled throughout hospitalization. It should be emphasized to the care team that MAT is for prevention of opioid withdrawal only and does NOT provide analgesia. Fetal monitoring may be altered by MAT, particularly methadone; decreased fetal movement and variability may occur for a few hours following a dose [7]. Because MAT medications have a long half-life, a short delay in medication administration can be appropriate if delivery will occur close to the time of usual administration. The partial opioid agonists nalbuphine (Nubain®) and butorphanol (Stadol®) are contraindicated in women with OUD, as they may precipitate withdrawal in the opioid-dependent patient [8, 9]. Pediatricians should be aware of opioid-exposed newborns to ensure assessment for neonatal withdrawal symptoms.

# Intrapartum Care for the Parturient with Opioid Use Disorder (OUD)

Below are recommendations for three common presentations of the parturient with OUD: excellent prenatal care and stable in MAT treatment; limited or no prenatal care but stable in MAT treatment; or no MAT treatment and currently using illicit opioids.

## Scenario 1: Patient has been Receiving Regular Prenatal Care and is in a Program with Medication Assisted Therapy (MAT) with Either Methadone or Buprenorphine

On admission, medications should be reviewed and the current MAT medication and dose verified and ordered. Ideally, this information would be current in the patient's prenatal record. While verification from the prescribing physician is optimal, it is not always feasible and patient report can be used. Daily MAT medication should be prescribed on schedule to avoid opioid withdrawal. If the patient has been providing regular urine drug screens that are readily available to the pediatric providers, this could be omitted.

## Scenario 2: Patient has been Noncompliant with Prenatal Care but is Well Established in an MAT Program

When pregnancy care and MAT care are not co-located, some obstetric patients are compliant with MAT but not obstetric care. It is important for MAT providers

to incorporate compliance with obstetric care into the MAT treatment plan and respond accordingly. Nonetheless, women will arrive in labor and delivery stating they have OUD-treated with MAT without other documentation. In this setting, management is similar to the approach to any patient lacking prenatal care, including rapid tests for infection. Medication and dose should be verified. If the patient arrives off hours, if they have been compliant with MAT the center could be called in the AM (if daily dosing) or pharmacy or prescription monitoring system used to verify dose and prescriber (buprenorphine). Medication assisted therapy should be prescribed on schedule to avoid opioid withdrawal. Urine drug screening at admission is indicated.

## Scenario 3: Patient Admits to Opioid Use Disorder at the Time of Arrival to Labor and Delivery; No Active Treatment

This scenario can be the most challenging. There are few studies in the literature to guide the optimal approach. A detailed history of opioid intake, frequency, and symptoms of withdrawal that the patient has experienced in the past can be helpful in predicting when the patient might experience withdrawal. Urine drug screen is required. Liver enzymes, renal function, and infectious disease screening should be performed at the time of admission (in addition to prenatal labs) due to the potential of exposure with illicit drug use. Assessment for opioid withdrawal should be performed throughout the entire hospitalization, using a tool familiar to the nursing staff such as COWS (see Chapter 11). Fetal monitoring should be initiated with evidence of withdrawal. Medication assisted therapy can be initiated with the medication that best fits the needs of the patient for longer term follow-up. Women taking illicit methadone may tolerate methadone better than buprenorphine due to precipitated withdrawal symptoms observed with methadone to buprenorphine transitions [10]. Methadone can be started at a dose of 10 mg, not to exceed 30 mg daily for the first 3–4 days due to the long half-life and risk of overdose with rapid escalation. Buprenorphine/naloxone may be the optimal medication in some settings when it is known that will be the available medication for post-delivery care. Buprenorphine initiation should follow the usual buprenorphine induction policies as detailed in Chapter 11; if patients are experiencing mild withdrawal symptoms, buprenorphine is not likely to precipitate opioid withdrawal symptoms. Buprenorphine can be started at dose of 2–4 mg and titrated as needed for symptoms. Regardless of medication choice, the goal of therapy is to prevent overt withdrawal during hospitalization; dose optimization can occur over the next days or as an outpatient.

## Intrapartum and Postpartum Pain Control

Pain during childbirth remains one of the most frequent concerns of pregnant women for good reason: there is no way to avoid some discomfort during the birth process. Pain is a physiological and psychological process, with processing of classic receptor mediated responses modulated by the emotional stress areas of the brain. As such, there is wide variability of pain perception, but almost all women report discomfort during labor and delivery.

Increased sensitivity to pain, both in pain threshold and perception, has been described in individuals with chronic opioid exposure. Both opioid tolerance (requirement of increased dose of medication for a similar effect) and opioid induced hyperalgesia (OIH, increased sensitivity to pain) may explain these observations [11]. OIH is not improved by MAT: individuals presenting for treatment for heroin dependence have increased pain perception that persists after the initiation of methadone or buprenorphine [12], though may be better with buprenorphine than methadone given partial agonist effects. The mechanism of increased pain perception with OIH is not completely understood, but involves alteration of anatomic (apoptosis of dorsal horn neurons) and neurotransmitter (NMDA, spinal dynorphin) pathways. Of these, the glutamate-activated NMDA pathway deserves specific attention. Pain starts as a peripheral stimulus, transmitted to the dorsal horn of the spinal cord. Here, glutamate activation of the NMDA receptor enhances the pain signal and can decrease the pain threshold and increase pain perception. Opioids can phosphorylate the NMDA receptor, increasing activation, and therefore increase pain sensitivity and perception; persistent pain stimuli can ramp up the NMDA pathway and lead to intractable pain that can occur in opioid-dependent individuals. Ketamine blocks this NMDA ramp up response, making it a valuable adjunctive analgesic as noted below.

It is a common misconception that women with OUD tolerate labor pain poorly. While there are no data in women with untreated OUD, women with adequate control of OUD with MAT (methadone or buprenorphine) appear to tolerate labor similarly to control women. Compared to control (non-OUD) women, patients with OUD stable on MAT (methadone or buprenorphine) present for admission with similar pain scores (on a scale of 1–10: methadone vs control: 5 vs 6.5; buprenorphine vs control: 4 vs 5.3), request parenteral opioids for analgesia at a similar rate (methadone vs control: 4.4 percent vs 6.5 percent; buprenorphine vs control: 4.5 percent vs 6.8 percent), and have a similar rate of delivery without analgesia (methadone versus control: 9 percent vs 11 percent; buprenorphine versus control: 13.6 percent vs 15.9 percent) [13, 14]. Women had similar high levels of pain before requesting regional analgesia (pain scores 9 out of 10 in all groups). Overall, these data confirm the high level of pain associated with labor for all women and similar rates of unmedicated childbirth regardless of OUD status. It is notable that there is no evidence of parenteral opioid-seeking behavior during labor.

## Interventions for Pain Control in Labor

There are multiple modalities for pain relief in labor, with variability in efficacy in the general population. These are discussed below, although our understanding of the efficacy in women with OUD is limited [15], except for neuraxial analgesia/anesthesia.

## Nonpharmacologic Interventions

Nonpharmacologic methods of pain control in labor include hypnosis, biofeedback, saline injections, immersion in water, aromatherapy, yoga, music, acupuncture, massage, and other stress reduction modalities. There is minimal to no effect on pain or obstetric outcome of each of these techniques when examined in routine laboring patients, although study design and control groups varied [15]. None of the nonpharmacologic therapies for pain control during labor have been specifically tested in the opioid-dependent population. These modalities leverage endogenous reward or stress reduction circuits, which are likely compromised in patients with OUD, and as such may be less effective for these women. Nonetheless, these modalities are safe, many are readily available in labor and delivery suites, and there is no reason not to offer any nonpharmacologic therapy to women with OUD as an option for pain control in labor. An added benefit of encouraging any of the techniques above in the labor and delivery setting is that women uninterested in trying nonpharmacologic relaxation at home can receive instruction in the hospital with an experienced nursing staff. In summary, many nonpharmacologic approaches are offered to all women in labor, and women with OUD should be offered the same instruction. Discussion of these options during the prenatal course can also empower women by providing choices. This is especially important for women who have been subject to trauma.

## Pharmacologic Interventions

### Inhaled Analgesia

Nitrous oxide ($N_2O$) is the only widely used inhaled analgesic used for labor pain management in the United States although other inhaled anesthetics have been studied: no study has been performed on women with OUD [15]. Inhalation is self-administered in subanesthetic doses, with common side effects of nausea, vomiting, and dizziness. Nitrous oxide does reduce the severity of pain in the first stage of labor; side effects may be dose-related. While the mechanism of action of inhaled analgesics is uncertain, it is likely regulated by endogenous opioid pathways and may be less effective in the opioid tolerant patient. The concurrent use of opioids and $N_2O$ can amplify respiratory depression effects of each. $N_2O$ in the patient with OUD should be administered with caution, with increased attention to the sedating effects of combined use, especially if methadone was recently administered. Given its limited efficacy in general and potential for increased risk, $N_2O$ is not an optimal choice for analgesia in the patient with OUD.

### Parenteral Opioids

Parenteral opioids, administered IM or IV, have been commonly used for management of early labor pain for many years with scant data. Use has been restricted to early labor due to the concern for respiratory depression in the neonate delivered soon after maternal opioid administration. In an effort to reduce the potential of neonatal respiratory depression, mixed agonist/antagonist medications (nalbuphine, butorphanol, tramadol) are commonly used instead of full opioid agonists (morphine). Both nalbuphine and butorphanol can precipitate opioid withdrawal in opioid-dependent individuals and should be considered contraindicated in women with OUD as was mentioned earlier [8, 9]. Indeed, the emergence of opioid withdrawal following

administration of one of the medications might alert the clinician to an undisclosed OUD; in this setting, rapid administration of a full opioid agonist will reverse withdrawal symptoms and restore maternal and fetal health (Figure 12.2). Although there are no trials comparing IV full agonist opioid to placebo for labor pain, it has been well established that full agonist opioids are effective for acute pain relief and can be considered in the management of early labor pain. Parenteral opioids for the management of acute pain should not be withheld from women with OUD, including labor pain. Because of the opioid tolerance of women with OUD, increased dosing may be required for pain relief.

### Neuraxial Analgesia for Labor

There is overwhelming acceptance that neuraxial analgesia, specifically epidural analgesia (sometimes combined with spinal) with low concentration local anesthetic (usually bupivacaine) and a small amount of opioid (usually fentanyl), is the most effective method of pain relief for severe labor and delivery pain. In labor and delivery settings with high rates of neuraxial analgesia use, there is no difference in use in women treated with MAT versus control women (methadone vs control: 80 percent vs 78 percent; buprenorphine vs control: 88 percent vs 82 percent) [13, 14]. In populations with a lower rate of neuraxial analgesia use, women treated with MAT had increased use of neuraxial analgesia use in labor compared to control women (MAT vs control: 38 percent vs 14 percent) [16], although whether there was bias against other options of labor analgesia for women on MAT (such as parenteral opioids or $N_2O$) was not addressed. Neuraxial analgesia is highly effective for labor and delivery pain control in women on MAT compared to controls. Women have high levels of pain when requesting neuraxial analgesia, regardless of MAT type or compared to control women (pain score 9 out of 10 for all groups) and have similarly excellent response to the initiation of analgesia (pain score 1–2 out of 10 for all groups). During labor, patient-controlled epidural analgesia (PCEA) with the standard epidural infusate (1/16 percent bupivacaine with 2 mcg/ml fentanyl) is effective, although adjustments in PCEA settings may be needed more frequently during labor. While there are no data on neuraxial analgesia for women with untreated OUD, this modality is still likely to be the most effective approach to intrapartum pain. It is of utmost importance that unexplained pain be assessed comprehensively, not

(a) Admission FHR: patient maintained on methadone

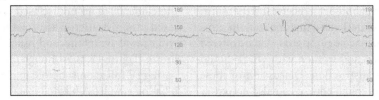

(b) Patient in acute withdrawal with fetal tachycardia following nalbuphine administration

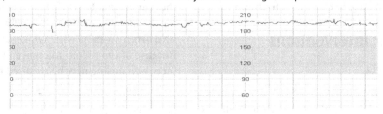

(c) Resolution of patient and fetal symptoms following IV morphine

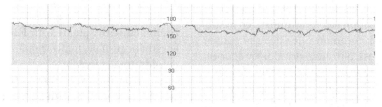

**Figure 12.2** (a) Fetal heart rate in a methadone maintained patient at the time of admission. (b) Following administration of nalbuphine 10 mg IV, fetal tachycardia occurs; the patient was symptomatic with severe withdrawal symptoms. (c) Following morphine IV with recovery of fetal heart rate to a normal baseline and normal variability, the patient's symptoms were improved

assumed to be related to OUD, as unrecognized uterine rupture or abruption can occur.

# Cesarean Delivery and Perioperative Medications

Multimodal anesthesia and analgesia – the use of multiple perioperative adjunctive medications – has improved postoperative pain control and can reduce opioid use in the general population [17]. Overall, efficacy of multimodal analgesia in the OUD population, with or without MAT, has been poorly studied. In general, adjunctive medications use non-opioid dependent pathways and are appropriate for use in the patient with OUD. Most cesarean deliveries in the United States are performed with neuraxial anesthesia using local anesthetic with short acting opioid (fentanyl). Both provide effective operative pain control for women on MAT, similar to control women [13, 14, 16]. Addition of an intrathecal opioid (fentanyl, morphine, hydromorphone) can improve post-operative pain control, but not without side effects, most notably pruritus and nausea. Pruritus is more common following cesarean delivery (compared to other surgical procedures), with an incidence of 80–100 percent. The only treatment for pruritus is naloxone infusion, which would be contraindicated in women with OUD, though some centers have used diphenhydramine 25–50 mg with variable symptomatic relief. Since relief from pruritus is not available to women with OUD and the benefit of improved pain control has not been well established in this population, the risks and benefits of long acting intrathecal morphine or hydromorphone should be carefully weighed; alternatives such as intrathecal fentanyl (which is shorter duration and less pruritic) or other adjunctive medications may be preferred.

Other perioperative medications include infusion of low-dose ketamine (an NMDA blocker that can reduce the pain ramp up), gabapentin or pregabalin (modulators of glutamate pain response), parenteral nonsteriodal anti-inflammatory medications (ketorolac), parental acetaminophen, and odansetron (improves nausea related to intrathecal opioids). Of these medications, low dose ketamine has the most potential to improve pain control in women with OUD due to the increased sensitivity to pain common

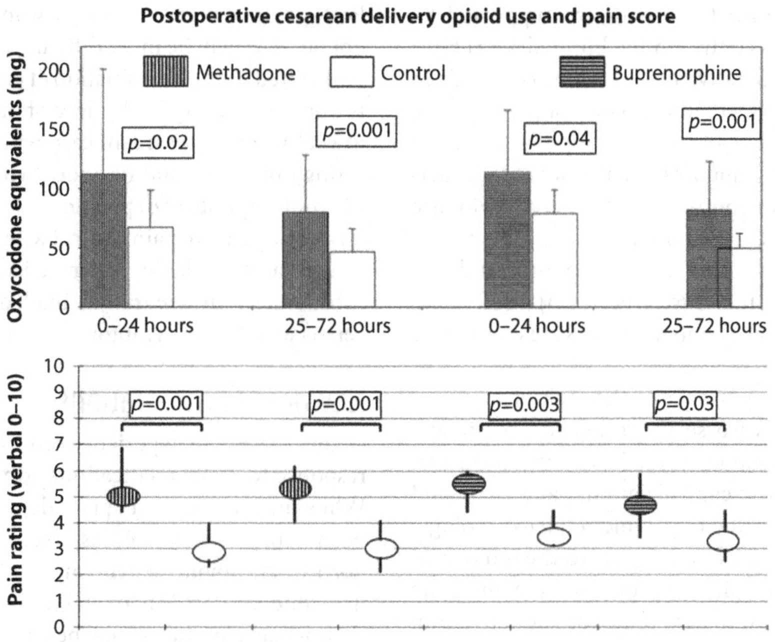

**Figure 12.3** Pain scores and oxycodone use in women treated with methadone or buprenorphine following cesarean delivery. Adapted from [12, 13].

with OUD via the NMDA system as described above; use of ketamine was shown to reduce opioid consumption following cesarean in nonopioid-dependent patients [18] and during lithotripsy in opioid-dependent patients [19], although no study has demonstrated improved pain control with cesarean delivery. Infiltration of the surgical area with local anesthetic, either within the incision or the tranversus abdominis plane block (TAP), can reduce postoperative pain and/or opioid requirements in the general population, but has not been reported specifically in patients with OUD [20]. Overall, the effects of each are modest and some are not synergistic: for example, the TAP block does not improve pain control over intrathecal morphine. Nonetheless, as individual postoperative pain treatment plans are developed with women undergoing cesarean delivery, adjunctive modalities should be considered.

## Postpartum Vaginal Birth

Pain following vaginal delivery is usually well controlled without opioid analgesics, but can increase with extensive lacerations. There are no data on women with uncontrolled OUD. Women maintained on methadone or buprenorphine both experienced higher pain

scores compared to control (pain scores 2.7 vs 1.5–2.0) but used similar amounts of oxycodone (10–12 mg vs 5–7 mg), ibuprofen, and acetaminophen [13, 14, 16]. There is no evidence that MAT type (methadone vs buprenorphine) has an impact on pain control post vaginal birth [21]. Overall, these data suggest that opioid use following vaginal birth is modest and can be offered on an as needed basis in the hospital; there is no evidence that opioid analgesics should be prescribed at discharge following uncomplicated vaginal delivery.

## Postpartum Cesarean Delivery

Treatment of acute pain in the opioid-tolerant patient is a challenge regardless of etiology. Multimodal interventions described above should be used liberally; the impact of multimodal therapies has not been tested in women with OUD, with or without MAT. The data we have for women on MAT versus control demonstrate increased pain and increased use of short acting opioids (Figure 12.3). Women on MAT require 50–70 percent more short-acting opioid following cesarean delivery, but decrease opioid use throughout the hospitalization similarly to control women. Although not directly compared, postoperative pain scores and opioid use are similar with women treated with methadone versus buprenorphine; these data are supported by the findings of pain control in the blinded MOTHER study, where postoperative opioid use was similar in women treated with methadone versus buprenorphine [21]. Use of ibuprofen and acetaminophen was similar. Overall, the data support higher doses of short acting opioids for pain control but there is no evidence that duration of therapy should be longer than control women (although this has been poorly studied). It is of note that all studies were performed before the multimodal approaches noted above were commonly employed.

Of particular importance is the lack of evidence that pain control is worse in women on buprenorphine versus methadone. There has been substantial concern of inability to control pain in patients treated with buprenorphine due to its unique pharmacologic profile: buprenorphine binds tightly to the mu opioid receptor, the major opioid receptor for the analgesic effect of opioids, but allows only partial activation. Theoretically, buprenorphine should block the actions of short acting opioids more effectively than the full mu opioid agonist, methadone. The relative equivalence of the opioid dosing and pain scores following cesarean delivery suggests the impact of short acting opioids and the mechanisms of opioid tolerance and pain modulation are similar for methadone and buprenorphine.

Discontinuation of buprenorphine in preparation for surgical procedures has been proposed as a mechanism for improved post-operative pain control. There are a number of reasons to avoid this approach:

1. With a cesarean rate close to 30 percent nationally, it is impossible to plan for a surgical procedure in a majority of the cesarean deliveries.
2. Cessation of buprenorphine, transition to short acting opioids for maintenance, then reintroduction of buprenorphine postpartum requires multiple stressful transitions at a vulnerable time for women and increases the risk for relapse with sequelae.
3. There are no data that support improved pain control following cesarean when compared to a long acting full mu opioid agonist (methadone). Finally, it has been demonstrated that pain can be controlled with increased doses of short acting opioid in the inpatient setting. There is no clear justification for changing MAT immediately around delivery for the purpose of improved pain control.

Postoperative pain control for women with OUD but not on MAT will be more difficult, as opioid needs will be dictated by the combination of pain and withdrawal. If women have required a dose of methadone for withdrawal prior to cesarean, care with additional short-acting opioids should be added with careful attention to avoid respiratory depression. Placement of epidural for post-operative pain control with patient-controlled analgesia, if available, is very effective and may help substantially in separating inadequate pain control versus withdrawal symptoms (Figure 12.4).

## Newborn Considerations

Neonates will not experience respiratory depression in response to MAT medications administered in labor. While the exact level of opioid dependence in the newborn cannot be reliably assessed at birth, no infant born to an opioid-dependent mother should receive naloxone as a part of neonatal resuscitation as neonatal abstinence symptoms may be precipitated. Naloxone administration has been removed from the most recent neonatal resuscitation guidelines.

## Breastfeeding

Methadone and buprenorphine (with or without naloxone) are compatible with breastfeeding. Breastfeeding has been associated with fewer neonatal abstinence symptoms and may improve maternal bonding. In the absence of a contraindication, mothers should be encouraged to breastfeed with the caveats explained in Chapter 15. Women with untreated OUD are still candidates for breastfeeding if they are starting MAT and can be observed in the hospital. Contraindications to breastfeeding include active use of cocaine or amphetamines and HIV infection; women with hepatitis C should still be encouraged to breastfeed in the absence of cracked, bleeding nipples.

## Patient Considerations

It is of note that the patients themselves may fear relapse in the setting of pain and prescribed opioids; some may have started opioid misuse in such a setting [11]. Patients with OUD may be afraid to be seen as drug seeking and have untreated pain as a result. Discussing the importance of adequate pain control with patients with OUD is important.

Opioid storage should be specifically addressed for all patients but especially with those with OUD, who may have a higher risk of medication loss. In a survey

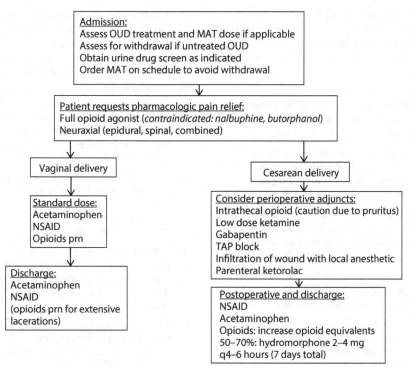

**Admission:**
Assess OUD treatment and MAT dose if applicable
Assess for withdrawal if untreated OUD
Obtain urine drug screen as indicated
Order MAT on schedule to avoid withdrawal

**Patient requests pharmacologic pain relief:**
Full opioid agonist (*contraindicated: nalbuphine, butorphanol*)
Neuraxial (epidural, spinal, combined)

Vaginal delivery

Cesarean delivery

**Standard dose:**
Acetaminophen
NSAID
Opioids prn

**Consider perioperative adjuncts:**
Intrathecal opioid (caution due to pruritus)
Low dose ketamine
Gabapentin
TAP block
Infiltration of wound with local anesthetic
Parenteral ketorolac

**Discharge:**
Acetaminophen
NSAID
(opioids prn for extensive lacerations)

**Postoperative and discharge:**
NSAID
Acetaminophen
Opioids: increase opioid equivalents
50–70%: hydromorphone 2–4 mg
q4–6 hours (7 days total)

**Figure 12.4** Algorithm for intrapartum and postpartum pain control in women with opioid use disorder treated with methadone or buprenorphine

of patients following cesarean delivery, 77 percent kept their prescribed short acting opioids in an unsecured location [22]. Physicians should take care to prescribe only the amount of short acting opioid needed and discuss the importance of locked medication storage.

# References

1. Boba A. Management of acute alcoholic intoxication. *The American Journal of Emergency Medicine* 1999;17:431.

2. Asplund C. A., Aaronson J. W., Aaronson H. E. 3 Regimens for alcohol withdrawal and detoxification. *Journal of Family Practice* 2004 July;53(7):545–54.

3. Kosten T. R., O'Connor P. G. Management of drug and alcohol withdrawal. *The New England Journal of Medicine* 2003;348:1786–96.

4. Weinbroum A. A., Flaishon R., Sorkine P., Szold O., Rudick V. A risk–benefit assessment of flumazenil in the management of benzodiazepine overdose. *Drug Safety* 1997;17:181–95.

5. Kawasaki S. S., Jacapraro J. S., Rastegar D. A. Safety and effectiveness of a fixed-dose phenobarbital protocol for inpatient benzodiazepine detoxification. *Journal of Substance Abuse Treatment* 2012;43:331–4.

6. Phillips K., Luk A., Soor G. S., et al. Cocaine cardiotoxicity: a review of the pathophysiology, pathology, and treatment options. *American Journal of Cardiovascular Drugs: Drugs, Devices, and Other Interventions* 2009;9:177–96.

7. Salisbury A. L., Coyle M. G., O'Grady K. E., et al. Fetal assessment before and after dosing with buprenorphine or methadone. *Addiction* 2012;107(Suppl 1):36–44.

8. Preston K. L., Bigelow G. E., Liebson I. A. Antagonist effects of nalbuphine in opioid-dependent human volunteers. *The Journal of Pharmacology and Experimental Therapeutics* 1989;248:929–37.

9. Preston K. L., Bigelow G. E., Liebson I. A. Butorphanol-precipitated withdrawal in opioid-dependent human volunteers. *The Journal of Pharmacology and Experimental Therapeutics* 1988;246:441–8.

10. Salsitz E. A., Holden C. C., Tross S., Nugent A. Transitioning stable methadone maintenance patients to buprenorphine maintenance. *Journal of Addiction Medicine* 2010;4:88–92.

11. Eyler E. C. Chronic and acute pain and pain management for patients in methadone maintenance treatment. *The American Journal on Addictions* 2013;22:75–83.

12. Compton P., Canamar C. P., Hillhouse M., Ling W. Hyperalgesia in heroin dependent patients and the effects of opioid substitution therapy. *The Journal of Pain: Official Journal of the American Pain Society* 2012;13:401–9.

13. Meyer M., Wagner K., Benvenuto A., Plante D., Howard D. Intrapartum and postpartum analgesia for women maintained on methadone during pregnancy. *Obstetrics and Gynecology* 2007;110:261–6.

14. Meyer M., Paranya G., Keefer Norris A., Howard D. Intrapartum and postpartum analgesia for women maintained on buprenorphine during pregnancy. *European Journal of Pain* 2010;14:939–43.

15. Jones L., Othman M., Dowswell T., et al. Pain management for women in labour: an overview of systematic reviews. *The Cochrane Database of Systematic Reviews* 2012;(3): Art. No. CD009234.

16. Hoflich A. S., Langer M., Jagsch R., et al. Peripartum pain management in opioid dependent women. *European Journal of Pain* 2012;16:574–84.

17. Gritsenko K., Khelemsky Y., Kaye A. D., Vadivelu N., Urman R. D. Multimodal therapy in perioperative analgesia. *Best Practice & Research. Clinical Anaesthesiology* 2014;28:59–79.

18. Behdad S., Hajiesmaeili M. R., Abbasi H. R., et al. Analgesic effects of intravenous ketamine during spinal aesthesia in pregnant women undergone caesarean section: a randomized clinical trial. *Anesthesiology and Pain Medicine* 2013;3:230–3.

19. Gharaei B., Jafari A., Aghamohammadi H., et al. Opioid-sparing effect of preemptive bolus low-dose ketamine for moderate sedation in opioid abusers undergoing extracorporeal shock wave lithotripsy: a randomized clinical trial. *Anesthesia and Analgesia* 2013;116:75–80.

20. Mishriky B. M., George R. B., Habib A. S. Transversus abdominis plane block for analgesia after Cesarean delivery: a systematic review and meta-analysis. *Canadian Journal of Anaesthesia – Journal Canadien D'anesthesie* 2012;59:766–78.

21. Jones H. E., O'Grady K., Dahne J., et al. Management of acute postpartum pain in patients maintained on methadone or buprenorphine during pregnancy. *The American Journal of Drug and Alcohol Abuse* 2009;35:151–6.

22. Bartels K., Mayes L. M., Dingmann C., et al. Opioid use and storage patterns by patients after hospital discharge following surgery. *PLoS One* 2016;11:e0147972.

# Postpartum Care for Women with Substance Use Disorders

Elizabeth E. Krans, Sebastian T. Tong and Mishka Terplan

## Introduction

The postpartum period is a critical transition for women with substance use disorders (SUD) and is characterized by significant physiologic, social and emotional change. Often referred to as the "fourth trimester," the postpartum period is traditionally defined as the 6–8-week period after delivery of the baby due to resolution of the physiological effects of pregnancy on maternal organ systems during this time [1]. However, because of the profound social, emotional and economic impact that pregnancy and childbirth have on many women, the postpartum transition is currently thought of as lasting up to 12 months after delivery [2].

Pregnancy is often characterized as a window of opportunity to provide preventative health care services. In contrast, the postpartum period presents multiple challenges and represents a period of unique vulnerability for women with SUD. Stresses associated with parenting, increased financial demands, limited resource availability and sleep deprivation can be overwhelming for women that often have limited social support [3]. Postpartum depression and anxiety, incomplete transitions from obstetric to primary care providers and loss of pregnancy-related insurance eligibility after delivery place women at significant risk of relapse and treatment discontinuation. Therefore, efforts to enhance care coordination among providers and increased attention to the complex psychiatric, social and environmental factors faced by women with SUD during the postpartum period can dramatically improve outcomes for this particularly vulnerable population [4].

## Substance Use, Relapse and Treatment Discontinuation

Pregnancy is associated with a reduction in substance use for the majority of women [5]. Over half of women who report pre-pregnancy tobacco use quit smoking prior to their first prenatal appointment [6]. Likewise, 90 percent of women abstain from alcohol use and 70–100 percent of women abstain from other substances including cannabis, prescription opioids, and cocaine during pregnancy [7, 8]. Time to abstinence during pregnancy is shortest for alcohol followed by cocaine, cannabis, and cigarettes, with most women achieving abstinence by the second trimester. When all substances are evaluated concurrently, over 80 percent of women discontinue the use of at least one substance during pregnancy [9].

Conversely, women often resume substance use in the postpartum period. According to the National Survey on Drug Use and Health (NSDUH), binge alcohol (10.0 percent vs. 1.0 percent), cigarette (20.4 percent vs. 13.9 percent), and cannabis use (3.8 percent vs. 1.4 percent) are significantly higher among women during the first 3 months postpartum when compared to the third trimester of pregnancy [5]. Resumption of substance use can occur rapidly as approximately half of women who quit smoking during pregnancy, resume within the first 2 weeks postpartum [10]. Women with opioid use disorder (OUD) who are on medication-assisted treatment (MAT) are also at significantly increased risk of treatment discontinuation in the postpartum period. In an evaluation of over 200 women with OUD on methadone, the estimated probability of methadone discontinuation before 6 months postpartum was 56 percent [11].

Postpartum relapse carries a heightened risk of overdose and overdose death. In contrast to global trends, the maternal mortality rate is increasing in the United States, related in part to the opioid epidemic [12]. From 2002 to 2011, the maternal mortality rate for substance use and overdose exceeded that of any obstetric cause (hemorrhage, emboli, preeclampsia, or sepsis) [13]. In Maryland, substance use and overdose was the leading cause of maternal death in 2015, with all deaths but one occurring in the postpartum period [14]. For this reason naloxone co-prescribing and overdose awareness education should be a routine part of postpartum care for women with OUD.

Multiple reasons may exist for resumption of substance use and treatment discontinuation in the postpartum period. First, the frequency and intensity of maternal health care utilization decreases significantly after pregnancy. Frequently, women with SUD receive a combination of care from prenatal care, SUD treatment and sometimes primary care providers. After delivery, women transition from seeing their obstetric care provider every week during the end of the third trimester to a single visit 4–6 weeks after delivery. There is a recalibration of health care providers following delivery and, as a result, the pediatrician is the health care provider that many women most frequently encounter postpartum. Second, communication is often limited, especially postpartum, between obstetricians and other health care providers, and between the inpatient and outpatient settings. Third, the traditional SUD treatment system is typically not designed to accommodate both women and their children. Only 40 percent of SUD treatment facilities in the United States offer any women-centered programming, 15 percent offer specific services for pregnant and postpartum women, and only 8 percent offer childcare [15]. Addressing some of these barriers to continued care may help prevent treatment discontinuation, relapse and overdose death, prolong abstinence and support recovery.

## Pain Management

Adequate control of pain in the immediate postpartum period can be challenging for women with OUD. Among women with OUD, acute pain is often underestimated and undertreated [16]. Furthermore, patients with a long history of OUD, including those who are prescribed methadone and/or buprenorphine, frequently have increased pain sensitivity and chronic hyperalgesia, especially after cesarean delivery [17]. In one small study, women who used methadone during their pregnancy required 70 percent more morphine milligram equivalents of opioids to adequately control their pain compared to women without OUD [17, 18]. Likewise, in another evaluation, women who used buprenorphine during pregnancy required 47 percent more opioids for pain control compared to those not on buprenorphine [19].

Given these challenges, special attention needs to be placed on adequate pain relief in the immediate postpartum period. Nonpharmacological interventions including abdominal binders, sitz-baths and analgesic sprays should be used as first-line therapy followed

by acetaminophen and anti-inflammatory medications, such as ibuprofen or ketorolac, for postpartum pain control. However, for those with inadequate pain control with these agents, short-acting opioids may be used in addition to continuation of maintenance doses of buprenorphine and methadone [20]. If women with OUD continue to require additional opioids for adequate pain relief, they should be prescribed the lowest effective dose of short-acting opioids for short durations, in accordance with the CDC opioid prescribing guidelines [21]. Judicious use of opioids combined with a prioritization of nonpharmacologic interventions and nonopioid medications can help promote compassionate, patient-centered care while protecting against opioid misuse.

## Breastfeeding

Breastfeeding and breastmilk may play a particularly beneficial role for women with OUD and their infants due to associations with decreased neonatal abstinence syndrome (NAS) severity, increased maternal confidence and enhanced maternal–child attachment [22–26]. In 2013, the American Academy of Pediatrics (AAP) emphasized the importance of breastfeeding for mothers on methadone or buprenorphine regardless of maternal dose. Despite recommendations, less than half of women who receive methadone pharmacotherapy breastfeed their infants after delivery. Even among women who breastfeed, up to 60 percent stop within 6 days of delivery [27]. However, OUD treatment programs that incorporate intensive prenatal and postpartum lactation counseling and support have shown far better breastfeeding initiation rates – 76 percent among women on buprenorphine [28]. In Guidelines for Breastfeeding and the Drug-Dependent Woman, breastfeeding recommendations for women with SUDs are clearly outlined [29]. Breastfeeding is not recommended for mothers who are actively using illicit drugs due to rapidly fluctuating levels of drug exposure.

## Contraception and Reproductive Health Care

Unintended pregnancy is common among women with SUDs [30, 31]. Over 86 percent of women with OUD report having an unintended pregnancy compared to 45 percent of the US population [30, 32]. Women with OUD also report a higher prevalence of rapid, repeat pregnancies with approximately one-third of women reporting six or more pregnancies [31]. In a survey of

183 women enrolled in opioid treatment programs, approximately half reported having their first pregnancy under the age of 18 and 57 percent of women reported ever having had an abortion, a rate that is twice that of the general population [31].

In evaluations of contraceptive use patterns of sexually active women with OUD, only 26–55 percent report using any form of contraception, despite the majority not wanting to get pregnant [31, 33–36]. When contraceptive method choice is evaluated, the majority of women report using condoms as their predominant form of contraception, with less than 10 percent reporting the use of high effective contraceptive methods also known as long acting reversible contraception (LARC) [33]. A lack of awareness about the effectiveness of different contraceptive methods, inadequate prenatal contraceptive counseling, and failure to provide highly effective contraceptive options in the immediate postpartum period are significant barriers to reducing unintended pregnancy in this population [37].

Pregnancy and the immediate postpartum period provide unique opportunities to provide comprehensive family planning counseling, education and services [38–40]. Enhanced patient engagement during pregnancy with both prenatal and SUD treatment providers can facilitate education and counseling regarding the effectiveness of available contraceptive methods, the importance of consistent condom use to prevent sexual transmitted infection and pregnancy planning. Long acting reversible contraception (LARC) such as intrauterine devices (IUDs) and subdermal implants are safe and highly effective in reducing the incidence of unintended pregnancy in all populations and should be encouraged over other methods due to significantly greater continuation rates when used for postpartum contraception [41, 42]. To further reduce the risk of unplanned pregnancy, immediate post-placental IUD placement or insertion of implants prior to discharge should also be considered [43]. Given that less than half of women enrolled in MAT programs attend the traditional postpartum appointment approximately 4–6 weeks after delivery emphasizes the importance of contraceptive planning and LARC utilization in the immediate postpartum period [44].

## Postpartum Mood Disorders

Women with SUD are more vulnerable to develop postpartum depression due to the high prevalence of co-occurring psychiatric disorders, limited social support, low self-esteem, and increased stress [45].

Emotional, physical and sexual abuse, which are also common among women with SUD, have also been consistently associated with an increased risk of postpartum depression [46]. The strongest risk factor for postpartum depression is a history of depression and the prevalence of co-occurring mood disorders such as depression, anxiety, bipolar disorder and posttraumatic stress disorder (PTSD) among women with OUD is estimated between 65 and 73 percent [47, 48]. Women with OUD and a co-occurring mood disorder are also at greater risk of adverse SUD treatment outcomes including both relapse and MAT discontinuation [48].

Approximately half of women with OUD screen positive for postpartum depression, a rate significantly higher than that of the general population [49]. As a result, all providers involved in the care of pregnant and postpartum women with SUDs should screen for perinatal depression. The most widely used screening tool used to identify depression in the postpartum period is the self-administered, 10-item Edinburgh Postnatal Depression Scale which takes less than 5 minutes to complete [50]. Screening for postpartum depression should occur at least once between 4 and 8 weeks after delivery, but may be administered more frequently for women with SUD [51]. Once depression is identified, the initiation of an antidepressant medication may be warranted. In particular, selective serotonin reuptake inhibitors (SSRI's) are safe and effective medications in the postpartum period and are compatible with breastfeeding [52].

## Social Support

Support from social workers, case managers, sponsors, and peer support groups such as narcotic anonymous (NA), alcoholics anonymous (AA) is critical to providing ongoing recovery support for women with a history of SUD after delivery. Many pregnant and postpartum women with SUD are at high risk for physical, emotional and sexual violence, have unstable or lack safe, drug-free housing, do not have reliable transportation and lack the financial resources necessary to provide for themselves and their children [53]. These social and environmental stressors are often exacerbated in the postpartum period when financial and emotional demands related to parenting and childcare are realized.

Special attention should be placed on communication between providers during the transition of care from the perinatal to postpartum period. Appropriate care for women with OUD will need to move beyond the traditional biomedical model to embrace a more holistic model of care. Much of the needed care may take place beyond the walls of the clinic and hospital. As such, systems that allow for adequate referral processes, integrated care and communication between providers will facilitate the successful care of postpartum women with OUD.

## Parenting

Perhaps the most important transition in the postpartum period is to the role of parent. Women with SUD face unique challenges related to caring for an infant that may need a prolonged hospitalization for complications related to prematurity and/or NAS. Once home from the hospital, chronically drug-exposed infants are more likely to have abnormal sleeping patterns, feeding difficulties and may be difficult to soothe due to overstimulation [54]. Moreover, many women with a history of SUD often have poor parental role modeling, have low self-esteem and inadequate coping mechanisms that may interfere with development of effective parenting skills [55]. In an evaluation of parenting knowledge among women in a drug treatment program, 64 percent of women wrongly believed that holding their baby when they cried would spoil them, 51 percent were not aware that holding their baby would result in less crying and 67 percent did not identify signs of infant stress [55]. In addition to limited parenting knowledge, 58 percent of women incorrectly believed that children exposed to drugs in utero were "born addicts" [55]. Women with SUD who are caring for children often feel stigmatized, which results in barriers to open conversations with pediatric providers and traditional support systems to help with parenting [56, 57]. As a result, parenting skills training and education should be an integral component of any program that provides care to pregnant and postpartum women with SUD.

## Child Welfare

State civil child-welfare statutes are heterogeneous in how they classify substance use during pregnancy. Currently 23 states and the District of Columbia consider substance use in pregnancy to be child abuse and 3 states consider it grounds for civil commitment [58]. The Child Abuse Prevention and Treatment Act (CAPTA) is one of the key pieces of federal legislation guiding child protection and the mechanism through which the federal government disburses block grants for local Department(s) of Social Services for child abuse and neglect prevention. Key elements of CAPTA include (1) the identification of infants born affected by substance use, withdrawal symptoms resulting from prenatal drug exposure or Fetal Alcohol Spectrum Disorder and (2) the establishment of a "Plan of Safe Care" for infants affected [59]. The Comprehensive Addiction and Recovery Act of 2016 additionally increased States' accountability by requiring, to the extent possible, reporting back to the federal government the number of infants identified as meeting the criteria in CAPTA and the number for whom a plan of safe care was developed. Consequentially, many states are considering legislation that would mandate notification to child protective services when these infants are born, in addition to the 7 states that currently mandate testing and the 23 states including the District of Columbia that currently mandate reporting [58]. Therefore, it is not uncommon for women with SUD to become involved with child welfare in the postpartum period which may result in child removal, maternal arrest, and the lifelong consequences of a child abuse conviction [60].

The consequence of the opioid epidemic on the child welfare system is profound. In 2014, a third of all child removals were due to parental alcohol or drug use compared to 14 percent in 1998, with the largest proportion of removals occurring during the first year [61]. While providers need to be aware of local reporting mandates and provide appropriate counseling to their patients, they should advocate for the dismantling of harmful legislation and for the expansion of treatment and associated services for women with SUD.

## Conclusions

Women with SUD face many challenges in the postpartum period. In addition to the physiologic, emotional and social changes that are faced by all postpartum women, those with SUD face additional barriers to appropriate care. These include stigma and discrimination, insufficient structural support for women who have children within the existing SUD treatment system, issues with adequate pain control, barriers to appropriate contraceptive management and breastfeeding support, and child welfare interference with care. Special attention to women with SUD in the postpartum period, including increased frequency of visits, intentionality of communication between providers and education about stigma may help reduce some of these issues and help support recovery and prevent relapse. Additional research to create evidence to promote policy changes to better support postpartum women with SUD will benefit both the health of the mother and the child.

# References

1. American Academy of Pediatrics, American College of Obstetricians and Gynecologists. *Guidelines for Perinatal Care*, 7th ed. 2012. http://simponline.it/wp-content/uploads/2014/11/GuidelinesforPerinatalCare.pdf

2. Committee on Obstetric P. The American College of Obstetricians and Gynecologists Committee opinion no. 630. Screening for perinatal depression. *Obstet Gynecol*. 2015;125(5):1268–71.

3. Gopman S. Prenatal and postpartum care of women with substance use disorders. *Obstet Gynecol Clin North Am*. 2014;41(2):213–28.

4. Jones H. E., Deppen K., Hudak M. L., et al. Clinical care for opioid-using pregnant and postpartum women: The role of obstetric providers. *Am J Obstet Gynecol*. 2014;210(4):302–10.

5. Substance Abuse and Mental Health Services Administration, Office of Applied Studies. The NSDUH Report: Substance Use among Women During Pregnancy and Following Childbirth. Rockville, MD, May 21, 2009.

6. Tong V. T., England L. J., Dietz P. M., Asare L. A. Smoking patterns and use of cessation interventions during pregnancy. *Am J Prev Med*. 2008;35(4):327–33.

7. Massey S. H., Lieberman D. Z., Reiss D., et al. Association of clinical characteristics and cessation of tobacco, alcohol, and illicit drug use during pregnancy. *Am J Addict*. 2011;20(2):143–50.

8. Tan C. H., Denny C. H., Cheal N. E., Sniezek J. E., Kanny D. Alcohol use and binge drinking among women of childbearing age – United States, 2011–2013. *MMWR – Morbid Mortal W*. 2015;64(37):1042–6.

9. Forray A., Merry B., Lin H., Ruger J. P., Yonkers K. A. Perinatal substance use: A prospective evaluation of abstinence and relapse. *Drug Alcohol Depend*. 2015;150:147–55.

10. Colman G. J., Joyce T. Trends in smoking before, during, and after pregnancy in ten states. *Am J Prev Med*. 2003;24(1):29–35.

11. Wilder C., Lewis D., Winhusen T. Medication assisted treatment discontinuation in pregnant and postpartum women with opioid use disorder. *Drug Alcohol Depend*. 2015;149:225–31.

12. MacDorman M. F., Declercq E., Cabral H., Morton C. Recent increases in the U.S. maternal mortality rate: Disentangling trends from measurement issues. *Obstet Gynecol*. 2016;128(3):447–55.

13. Koch A. R., Rosenberg D., Geller S. E. Higher risk of homicide among pregnant and postpartum females aged 10–29 years in Illinois, 2002–2011. *Obstet Gynecol*. 2016;128(3):440–6.

14. Maryland Department of Health and Mental Hygiene Prevention and Health Promotion Administration. Maryland Maternal Mortality Review: 2015 Annual Report, 2015.

15. Terplan M., Longinaker N., Appel L. Women-centered drug treatment services and need in the United States, 2002–2009. *Am J Public Health*. 2015;105(11):e50–4.

16. Mehta V., Langford R. M. Acute pain management for opioid dependent patients. *Anaesthesia*. 2006;61(3):269–76.

17. Compton P., Charuvastra V. C., Ling W. Pain intolerance in opioid-maintained former opiate addicts: Effect of long-acting maintenance agent. *Drug Alcohol Depend*. 2001;63(2):139–46.

18. Meyer M., Wagner K., Benvenuto A., Plante D., Howard D. Intrapartum and postpartum analgesia for women maintained on methadone during pregnancy. *Obstet Gynecol*. 2007;110(2 Pt 1):261–6.

19. Jones H. E., Johnson R. E., Milio L. Post-cesarean pain management of patients maintained on methadone or buprenorphine. *Am J Addict*. 2006;15(3):258–9.

20. Jones H. E., O'Grady K., Dahne J., et al. Management of acute postpartum pain in patients maintained on methadone or buprenorphine during pregnancy. *Am J Drug Alcohol Abuse*. 2009;35(3):151–6.

21. Dowell D. H. T., Chou R. CDC guideline for prescribing opioids for chronic pain – United States, 2016. *MMWR Recomm Rep* 2016;65(No. RR-1):1–49. DOI: http://dx.doi.org/10.15585/mmwr.rr6501e1.

22. Kocherlakota P. Neonatal abstinence syndrome. *Pediatrics*. 2014;134(2):e547–61.

23. Jansson L. M., Velez M., Harrow C. Methadone maintenance and lactation: A review of the literature and current management guidelines. *J Hum Lact Off J Int Lact Consult Assoc*. 2004;20(1):62–71.

24. Demirci J. R., Bogen D. L., Klionsky Y. Breastfeeding and methadone therapy: The maternal experience. *Subst Abuse Off Publication Assoc Med Educ Res Subst Abuse*. 2015;36(2):203–8.

25. Abdel-Latif M. E., Pinner J., Clews S., et al. Effects of breast milk on the severity and outcome of neonatal abstinence syndrome among infants of drug-dependent mothers. *Pediatrics*. 2006;117(6):e1163–9.

26. Jansson L. M., Choo R., Velez M. L., et al. Methadone maintenance and breastfeeding in the neonatal period. *Pediatrics*. 2008;121(1):106–14.

27. Wachman E. M., Byun J., Philipp B. L. Breastfeeding rates among mothers of infants with neonatal abstinence syndrome. *Breastfeed Med.* 2010;5(4): 159–64.

28. O'Connor A. B., Collett A., Alto W. A., O'Brien L. M. Breastfeeding rates and the relationship between breastfeeding and neonatal abstinence syndrome in women maintained on buprenorphine during pregnancy. *J Midwifery Wom Heal.* 2013;58(4):383–8.

29. Academy of Breastfeeding Medicine Protocol C, Jansson L. M. ABM clinical protocol #21: Guidelines for breastfeeding and the drug-dependent woman. *Breastfeed Med Off J Acad Breastfeed Med.* 2009;4(4):225–8.

30. Heil S. H., Jones H. E., Arria A., et al. Unintended pregnancy in opioid-abusing women. *J Subst Abuse Treat.* 2011;40(2):199–202.

31. Black K. I., Stephens C., Haber P. S., Lintzeris N. Unplanned pregnancy and contraceptive use in women attending drug treatment services. *Australian N Z J Obstet Gynaecol.* 2012;52(2):146–50.

32. Finer L. B., Zolna M. R. Declines in unintended pregnancy in the United States, 2008–2011. *N Eng J Med.* 2016;374(9):843–52.

33. Terplan M., Hand D. J., Hutchinson M., Salisbury-Afshar E., Heil S. H. Contraceptive use and method choice among women with opioid and other substance use disorders: A systematic review. *Prev Med.* 2015;80:23–31.

34. Morrison C. L., Ruben S. M., Beeching N. J. Female sexual health problems in a drug dependency unit. *Int J STD & AIDS.* 1995;6(3):201–3.

35. Ralph N., Spigner C. Contraceptive practices among female heroin-addicts. *Am J Public Health.* 1986;76(8):1016–7.

36. Cornford C. S., Close H. J., Bray R., Beere D., Mason J. M. Contraceptive use and pregnancy outcomes among opioid drug-using women: A retrospective cohort study. *PLoS One.* 2015;10(3). http://journals .plos.org/plosone/article?id=10.1371/journal. pone.0116231.

37. Terplan M., Lawental M., Connah M. B., Martin C. E. Reproductive health needs among substance use disorder treatment clients. *J Addict Med.* 2016;10(1):20–5.

38. Zapata L. B., Murtaza S., Whiteman M. K., et al. Contraceptive counseling and postpartum contraceptive use. *Am J Obstet Gynecol.* 2015;212(2).

39. Teal S. B. Postpartum contraception: Optimizing interpregnancy intervals. *Contraception.* 2014;89(6):487–8.

40. de Bocanegra H. T., Chang R., Howell M., Darney P. Interpregnancy intervals: Impact of postpartum

contraceptive effectiveness and coverage. *Am J Obstet Gynecol.* 2014;210(4):311.e1–8.

41. Parks C., Peipert J. F. Eliminating health disparities in unintended pregnancy with long-acting reversible contraception (LARC). *Am J Obstet Gynecol.* 2016;214(6):681–8.

42. Sinha C., Guthrie K. A., Lindow S. W. A survey of postnatal contraception in opiate-using women. *Journal Family Plan Reprod Health Care/Fac Family Plan Reprod Health Care, R Coll Obstet Gynaecol.* 2007;33(1):31–4.

43. Krans E. E., Dunn S. L. Health care use patterns of opioid-dependent pregnant women. *Obstet Gynecol.* 2014;123(Suppl 1):61S.

44. Parlier A. B., Fagan B., Ramage M., Galvin S. Prenatal care, pregnancy outcomes, and postpartum birth control plans among pregnant women with opiate addictions. *South Med J.* 2014;107(11):676–83.

45. Chapman S. L. C., Wu L. T. Postpartum substance use and depressive symptoms: A review. *Women Health.* 2013;53(5):479–503.

46. Ross L. E., Dennis C. L. The prevalence of postpartum depression among women with substance use, an abuse history, or chronic illness: A systematic review. *J Womens Health.* 2009;18(4):475–86.

47. Benningfield M. M., Arria A. M., Kaltenbach K., et al. Co-occurring psychiatric symptoms are associated with increased psychological, social, and medical impairment in opioid dependent pregnant women. *Am J Addict.* 2010;19(5):416–21.

48. Fitzsimons H. E., Tuten M., Vaidya V., Jones H. E. Mood disorders affect drug treatment success of drug-dependent pregnant women. *J Subst Abuse Treat.* 2007;32(1):19–25.

49. Holbrook A., Kaltenbach K. Co-occurring psychiatric symptoms in opioid-dependent women: The prevalence of antenatal and postnatal depression. *Am J Drug Alcohol Ab.* 2012;38(6):575–9.

50. Cox J. L., Holden J. M., Sagovsky R. Detection of postnatal depression – development of the 10-Item Edinburgh postnatal depression scale. *Brit J Psychiat.* 1987;150:782–6.

51. O'Connor E., Rossom R. C., Henninger M., Groom H. C., Burda B. U. Primary care screening for and treatment of depression in pregnant and postpartum women evidence report and systematic review for the US preventive services task force. *JAMA – J Am Med Assoc.* 2016;315(4):388–406.

52. Susser L. C., Sansone S. A., Hermann A. D. Selective serotonin reuptake inhibitors for depression in pregnancy. *Am J Obstet Gynecol.* 2016;215(6):722–30.

53. Young J. L., Martin P. R. Treatment of opioid dependence in the setting of pregnancy. *Psychiatric Clin North Am.* 2012;35(2):441–60.

54. Effects of in Utero Exposure to Street Drugs. *Am J Public Health*. 1993;83(Suppl):1–32.

55. Velez M. L., Jansson L. M., Montoya I. D., et al. Parenting knowledge among substance abusing women in treatment. *J Subst Abuse Treat*. 2004;27(3):215–22.

56. Wiig E. M., Halsa A., Haugland B. S. M. Social support available for substance-dependent mothers from families with parental substance abuse. *Child Family Soc Work*. 2016;211–26.

57. Stringer K. L., Baker E. H. Stigma as a barrier to substance abuse treatment among those with unmet need an analysis of parenthood and marital status. *J Family Issues*. 2015;1–25: doi: 10.11770192513X15581659.

58. The Guttmacher Institute. Substance Abuse During Pregnancy. Guttmacher Institute; 2017. Available from: www.guttmacher.org/state-policy/explore/substance-abuse-during-pregnancy

59. U.S. Department of Health and Human Services. *The Child Abuse Prevention and Treatment Act*. U.S. Department of Health and Human Services. Washington, DC, 2010.

60. Terplan M., Minkoff H. Neonatal abstinence syndrome and ethical approaches to the identification of pregnant women who use drugs. *Obstet Gynecol*. 2017;129(1):164–7.

61. U.S. Department of Health and Human Services. Adoption and Foster Care Analysis and Reporting System (AFCARS) Report #23. U.S. Department of Health and Human Services. 2016.

# Neonatal Abstinence Syndrome

Karol Kaltenbach and Loretta Finnegan

## History of Neonatal Abstinence Syndrome

The first surviving records of opium addiction date from the end of the eighteenth century although there are accounts of opium use from many centuries before that [1]. Morphine was isolated in 1804 and heroin was synthesized in 1874 [2]. Addiction to heroin and morphine became more common after their commercial production. As early as the nineteenth century [3], an increase in the incidence of morphine and heroin addiction among women was reported. Common thinking was that infants were not affected because morphine use among women was associated with sterility and a loss of sexual desire. In 1875, this was proven to be false after a case in a neonate who manifested signs of opioid withdrawal at birth was reported [4]. The diagnosis made was Congenital Morphinism and this case was followed by a number of similar reports [5], but sadly, most of the in-utero-exposed infants died after no specific treatment was offered [6]. In 1894, a series of 12 infants with Congenital Morphinism were treated with paregoric and 9 died. It is suspected that most of the infants died from prematurity and its complications as well as the lack of treatment for opioid withdrawal. In 1903, a report described an infant who survived after being treated with morphine [7]. When the successful treatment of seizures in an infant exposed to morphine in utero was reported in 1947 [8], Congenital Morphinism no longer was considered a medical curiosity. With the appearance of more reports [9, 10] significant attention to the condition occurred from obstetricians and pediatricians. Congenital Morphinism was subsequently renamed Neonatal Abstinence Syndrome (NAS) because of the constellation of signs culminating in one disease process.

Recently, the FDA has used the term neonatal opioid withdrawal syndrome (NOWS) when referring to maternal use of opioids during pregnancy with an outcome of withdrawal in the infant. However, there is some concern that this term is misplaced for use in a clinical setting. When NAS occurs as a result of prenatal exposure to an opioid, it occurs in a number of different contexts and the presentation and severity is related to a number of factors in addition to the opioid(s). Accordingly, this chapter will use the NAS terminology.

Between 1953 and 1955, 18 infants were reported with NAS. There was a 25 percent mortality rate due to prematurity and respiratory failure. The NAS was treated with methadone, phenobarbital, or paregoric. In 1956, 32 babies with NAS were reported with a 50 percent prematurity rate and a 34–93 percent mortality. When methadone was introduced for treating opioid addiction, it was thought that NAS would not occur [11]; however, it did and generally was more severe than that associated with heroin [12]. This could have been anticipated since patients received a steady dose of the medication whereas heroin doses on the street were variable.

Burgeoning numbers of babies with NAS were presenting to large city hospitals and reports by Blinick [13] and Zelson [14] from New York described the observed signs and the treatment that they were using, i.e., chlorpromazine [14]. Case series continued to be reported and then in 1975, Desmond and Wilson published a comprehensive paper on recognition and diagnosing NAS.

In 1974, realizing the need for research in the area of drug abuse in general and in perinatal drug dependence specifically, the Federal Government established the National Institute on Drug Abuse (NIDA) within the Alcohol Drug Abuse Mental Health Administration (ADAMHA). Areas researched included maternal medical effects on pregnancy and the newborn, psychological, and sociological aspects of maternal addiction, and comprehensive services for mother and the newborn. Many improvements in diagnosing and treating the maternal/infant dyad were established as a result of NIDA (now at NIH) funding. Recognizing that an assessment tool was important, in 1975, Finnegan et al. [15] (The Neonatal Abstinence Syndrome Score) and Lipsitz [16] (The Neonatal Withdrawal Scoring System) published their respective scoring tools.

Buprenorphine was approved in Europe in 1996 and in the United States in 2002 and NAS was found to be associated with this medication as well [17–20]. Neonatal abstinence associated with maternal use of prescription pain medications is included in the cases currently reported [21, 22]. Some of these opioid prescriptions and their date of reaching the marketplace include Percocet* (1976), Vicodin* (1984), and Oxycontin* (1996). The numbers of cases continued to escalate and have reached epidemic proportions in the past 10 years.

## Incidence of NAS

Historically, the incidence of NAS has been described in terms of the percentage of infants prenatally exposed to opioids who required treatment for NAS. These data are all based on cohort studies with a wide range of percentages reported, i.e. from 29 percent to as high as 94 percent [22, 23]. Such a wide range is often due to a lack of consistent operational definitions, either in clinical settings or research findings, when NAS is reported. Some restrict the diagnosis of NAS to when treatment is required; others base the diagnosis on any reported signs. Moreover, there are numerous factors, in addition to prenatal opioid exposure, that contribute to severity of withdrawal and are described in other sections within this chapter.

Within the past 5 years, numerous researchers have utilized national and state data sets based on IDC-9 hospital codes of neonatal drug withdrawal [24]. The initial study published in 2012 found that the incidence of NAS had increased almost fivefold from 2000 to 2009 [25]. Subsequent studies have found that the incidence varies significantly between states [26], that the geographic variations in NAS are consistent with the variations in opioid pain prescriptions [27], and that the incidence of NAS and maternal opioid use increased disproportionately in rural counties relative to urban counties [28]. While this research has helped to emphasize consequences of the current prescription opioid epidemic, there are many limitations to these data, specifically in relation to whether or not the infant required treatment. Additionally, these data do not differentiate NAS that occurs from illicit opioid use, e.g. drugs such as heroin and misuse

of prescription opioids, and NAS subsequent to appropriate maternal use of opioids under a physician's care, e.g. medication for treatment for opioid use disorder or pain management. While the risk of NAS may be comparable, the overall risk to the fetus and neonate may differ significantly.

## Morbidity in Infants Exposed to Opioids In Utero

Reports during the 1970s and 1980s showed that newborns of women using heroin had low birth weight and prematurity as the two most prominent medical issues. Conditions such as asphyxia neonatorum (respiratory failure due to inadequate intake of oxygen before, during, or just after birth), intracranial hemorrhage, nutritional deprivation, hypoglycemia (low blood sugar), hypocalcemia (low blood calcium), septicemia (bloodborne infection), and hyperbilirubinemia (jaundice) should also be anticipated in heroin-exposed babies. Infants exposed to methadone in utero are more likely to have higher birth weights and a decreased incidence of premature birth. Medical issues in infants born to women using heroin are generally influenced by the following: amount of prenatal care received by the mother; whether the mother suffered obstetrical or medical complications during the pregnancy; and whether the fetus was exposed to multiple drugs which can produce an unstable intrauterine milieu that can be further complicated by symptoms of withdrawal and overdose in both the woman and the fetus [29]. A number of reports [30, 31] demonstrate differences in heroin versus methadone exposed babies with regard to birth weight, neonatal problems, length of hospital stays, premature birth, and mortality. Rorke performed careful neuropathological examinations on preterm heroin-exposed babies whose mothers did not attend prenatal care or addictions services. She found lesions in the brains of the babies which demonstrated the result of hypoxia which probably occurred during maternal episodes of withdrawal or overdose, causing a lack of oxygen to the fetal brains [32].

It must be noted that data are lacking regarding morbidity in infants exposed to opioid pain medications. It is also unclear how morbidities differ in the contemporary population of infants born to women using illicit drugs. Some evidence is provided by Holbrook et al. [33] in which obstetric and neonatal outcomes in pregnant women with opioid use disorder (OUD) maintained on methadone or buprenorphine were examined. In a sample of 131 pregnant women with a history of heroin use or prescription misuse, the incidence of infectious medical complications and obstetric complications were much lower than historically reported rates among heroin users. Of import is that morbidity and mortality rates in pregnancy and in newborns can be decreased if women enroll in medication assisted treatment (MAT), receive prenatal care, and receive comprehensive services for the OUD [34].

## NAS and Concomitant Drug Use

Signs similar to opioid withdrawal in neonates have been described for alcohol, benzodiazepines, and Selective Serotonin Reuptake Inhibitors (SSRIs) [35]. While not all require treatment, the interaction of non-opioids and opioids can affect the presentation of NAS. SSRIs and benzodiazepines have consistently been found to contribute to NAS severity.

Studies have found SSRIs to be related to both the presentation and treatment of NAS, with higher peak scores of NAS [36] and higher doses of medication required for treatment [36, 37]. However, the concomitant use of SSRIs with opioids has not been found to predict whether infants would require treatment for NAS or length of treatment [36–39]. It should be emphasized that in the case of a pregnant woman requiring medication treatments for OUD and depression, these data should not be used to support treating one disorder over the other.

A number of studies have found benzodiazepines to be associated with prolonged length of stay in infants being treated for prenatal opioid exposure [38, 40, 41]. Benzodiazepine use and misuse is prevalent among pregnant women with opioid use disorders and presents both a risk to the fetus from maternal overdose sedation and possible death, and to the neonate from NAS that requires lengthy pharmacotherapy with multiple drugs.

Cigarette smoking in women with opioid use disorders has also been found to affect the timing and length of treatment of NAS [42, 43] as well as the total amount of medication required to treat NAS [43]. With appropriate medical management and/or behavioral intervention, the impact of benzodiazepines and cigarettes on NAS can be avoided.

A caveat must be included for this section in that all of the data that support the information provided here are derived from infants prenatally exposed to methadone or buprenorphine. This information may or may not be generalizable to other opioids.

## Variability in the Expression of NAS

In addition to concomitant drug use, there are several other factors related to the presentation of NAS. The gestational age of the infant has been found to be related to NAS with preterm infants requiring less treatment. One study found no difference in the need for treatment but it was the only study that limited the preterm group to late preterm, i.e. 34–36 weeks [44]. Studies have consistently found that preterm infants require less medication for treatment of NAS and have shorter duration of treatment [44–47]. Reasons for differences in opioid withdrawal for preterm infants are unknown with several possible explanations: (a) an immature hepatic metabolic system resulting in a gradual decline in serum concentration, (b) the developmental immaturity of the brain and associated opiate receptors, (c) less exposure over time to opioids, and (d) increased placental transfer of opioids in the third trimester [47]. It should be noted that all but one of these studies used the Finnegan Scoring Tool to assess NAS. The Finnegan tool was validated only for term infants and the use of this tool for preterm infants has not been validated. A validated NAS assessment for preterm infants may yield different results.

For decades, NAS due to prenatal opioid exposure was primarily the result of maternal heroin use and/or treatment with methadone for maternal OUD. With the addition of buprenorphine for the treatment of OUD, questions arose as to whether the frequencies of signs of NAS differ between the two medications. Data from the MOTHER study [48] were used to compare the NAS profile based on the MOTHER NAS (MNS) scale before treatment or in the absence of treatment in infants prenatally exposed to methadone or buprenorphine. The incidence of nasal stuffiness, sneezing, and loose stools was greater in the buprenorphine-exposed infants than the methadone-exposed infants. Additionally, methadone-exposed infants had higher mean scores for hyperactive Moro, disturbed and undisturbed tremors, failure to thrive, and excessive irritability [49]. Differences may exist between the two medications because of their pharmacological characteristics (full agonist versus partial agonist). These findings help explain differences in NAS severity between methadone and buprenorphine. There are no studies that have examined the NAS profile of infants prenatally exposed to opioid pain medications such as oxycodone, hydrocodone.

Several investigators have posited that the sex of the infant might play a role in predicting NAS severity since past studies have shown an increased vulnerability to adverse outcomes among males. Unger and colleagues [50], looking at sex-based differences in birth weight and length, head circumference, and NAS duration and severity, found that while males had a significantly higher birth weight and head circumference, there were no significant sex-related differences for NAS development, severity, duration, or medication administered. They reported that a similar postnatal vulnerability exists for both males and females, suggesting that factors other than sex are the major determinants of clinically significant NAS. No differences were found by Holbrook and Kaltenbach [51] in male versus female newborns with regard to the need for NAS treatment, length of treatment and peak dose of medication required.

Within the past 4 years, there has been significant, albeit preliminary, research to identify genetic and epigenetic factors that contribute to NAS variability. A series of studies from the same lab have progressively identified variants in the OPRMI and COMT genes associated with shorter length of hospital stay and less need for treatment in infants with NAS [52]; increased methylation within the OPRMI promoter associated with length of stay and the need for more than 2 medications to treat NAS [53]; and PNOC variants associated with NAS severity [54]. This work has exciting potential to provide individualized treatment regimens tailored specifically for infants with high-risk genetic profiles.

## NAS and Agonist Treatment for Opioid Use Disorders

Questions often arise regarding the use of MAT for opioid use disorders during pregnancy due to the expected occurrence of NAS. However, the risk to the infant for withdrawal is considered much less harmful than the benefits of MAT for the mother and fetus. The 1993 and 2004 SAMHSA Treatment Improvement Protocols for Opioid Use Disorders, the 1997 NIH Consensus Panel on Effective Medical Treatment of Opioid Addiction, the 2012 American College of Obstetricians and Gynecologists and American Society of Addiction Medicine Joint Opinion, the WHO 2014 Guidelines for the Identification and Management of Substance Use and Substance Use Disorders in Pregnancy and the 2016 SAMHSA Collaborative Approach to the

Treatment of Pregnant Women with Opioid Use Disorders all recommend MAT for pregnant women as the standard of care. Medications used to treat opioid use disorders in women who are pregnant are methadone, buprenorphine, and buprenorphine with naloxone (see Chapter 10 for a discussion on the use of these medications).

The relationship between maternal medication dose and NAS is often a question of clinicians, with the expectation that lower maternal medication dose will result in less severe NAS. This is especially applicable to methadone because of studies in the 1970s that recommended pregnant women be maintained on very low doses. An extensive literature from 1966 to 2009 was the subject of a systematic review and meta-analysis that found the severity of NAS does not differ between mothers on high or low doses of methadone [55]. A more recent study [56] examined the relationship between maternal methadone dose at delivery and neonatal outcomes with data from the MOTHER study and also found no relationship between maternal methadone dose and severity of NAS. These data are important to note because other drugs of abuse did not confound the sample and those who conducted the NAS assessment were trained to a gold standard of inter-rater reliability.

Due to buprenorphine's more recent approval, there is less literature on the relationship between maternal buprenorphine dose and severity of NAS. However, the available literature consistently reports no relationship. This includes a study with data from the MOTHER study that has the unique strengths mentioned above [57].

Differences in NAS as a function of whether the infant has been exposed to methadone or buprenorphine have been reported in a number of studies. The most widely referenced study is the MOTHER multisite randomized controlled trial [48]. This study ($n = 131$) found no difference in the number of infants in each medication group that required treatment for NAS. However, infants prenatally exposed to buprenorphine ($n = 58$) required 89 percent less morphine to treat NA, spent 58 percent less time in the hospital being medicated for NAS, and spent 43 percent less time in the hospital overall than infants prenatally exposed to methadone ($n = 73$). A systematic review and meta-analysis of 12 studies, including the MOTHER study, found similar results in that NAS treatment duration was shorter and morphine dose lower for buprenorphine-exposed infants than methadone-exposed infants [58].

While NAS outcomes are superior with buprenorphine than methadone, practitioners should not use that as the sole criteria for which medication to use during pregnancy. As a partial agonist, buprenorphine may not be effective for certain women and methadone may be the medication of choice for those women (refer to Chapter 10). Current recommendations suggest that women maintained on methadone or buprenorphine who become pregnant should remain on their respective medications. A pregnant woman who becomes pregnant who is naive to agonist treatment may be a good candidate for buprenorphine. If she does not respond well to buprenorphine she can easily be transitioned to methadone. Overall, the woman's medical, psychological, and substance use history should be taken into consideration in any treatment decision [59].

# NAS Onset and Signs

Infants with in utero exposure to opioids have a chance to be born with NAS. Reported percentages differ with the population studied. Psychoactive drugs, such as opioids, have low molecular weights and lipid solubility which permits them to pass easily from the mother to the fetus through the placenta. Once the drugs accumulate in the fetus, equilibrium is established between the maternal and fetal blood. When the umbilical cord is cut at birth, there is a disruption of the trans-placental passage of drugs potentially permitting the development of signs of abstinence. Affecting the central nervous, autonomic nervous, gastrointestinal, and respiratory systems, this constellation of signs constitutes the multisystem disorder called Neonatal Abstinence Syndrome. NAS can be a serious medical condition because it affects the vital functions that permit growth and normalcy in the newborn, i.e., feeding, elimination, and sleep. If untreated, NAS can cause death as was noted in the historical accounts. Death can occur because of excess fluid loss, high temperatures, seizures, respiratory instability, and aspiration of fluid into the lungs with cessation of breathing. Current medical knowledge about drug use during pregnancy and newborn care eliminates the chance of death from NAS [60].

Neonatal abstinence resulting from opioids is characterized by signs of CNS hyperirritability, gastrointestinal dysfunction, and respiratory and autonomic nervous system signs.

Central nervous system – Tremors, high pitched crying, hypertonia, irritability, increased deep tendon reflexes and an exaggerated startle reflex are all characteristics of neonatal abstinence. An exaggerated rooting reflex and a voracious appetite manifested as sucking of fists or thumbs are also common, yet when feedings are administered the infant may have extreme difficulty because of an uncoordinated sucking and swallowing mechanism. Kron et al. [61] found that both heroin and methadone-exposed infants showed reductions in sucking rates and pressures, disordered sucking organization and a reduction in the amounts of nutrient consumed. As a result of these issues, an infant affected by NAS may have difficulty during feeding. Breastfeeding can be challenging because of their disorganized sucking reflex but with support it can be accomplished. Seizures, a serious sign, fortunately occur infrequently. However, because they may be subtle or confused with exaggerated tremors, the reported incidence of seizures varies, ranging from 1 percent [60] to 5.9 percent [62] and 7.8 percent [63] of newborns exposed to heroin or methadone during pregnancy. Certain practices used in the treatment of NAS, such as tightly swaddling the infant in a darkened room, can also make it difficult to observe seizure movements.

Gastrointestinal system – Regurgitation, projectile vomiting, and loose stools are gastrointestinal manifestations of NAS. Dehydration because of poor intake, coupled with increased losses from the gastrointestinal tract, can cause excessive weight loss, electrolyte imbalance, shock, coma, and even death, however with current neonatal practices, this should not occur. Babies with mild NAS not requiring treatment can lose about 4 percent of their birth weight, regaining it by the 7th day of life. Newborns displaying more severe abstinence lose more weight and do not regain their weight until an average of 2 weeks after birth, suggesting that timely and appropriate pharmacological control of abstinence, combined with the provision of extra fluids and calories to offset the weight loss, are important in the management of NAS [64]. Although babies that exhibit mainly gastrointestinal symptoms might not meet the criteria for pharmacological treatment of their NAS, it is still extremely important for these babies to be monitored following discharge from the hospital because of the potential for water losses and poor intake, both of which can lead to dehydration.

Respiratory system – Increased respiratory rate can be accompanied by retractions between the ribs of the chest wall, intermittent cyanosis, and apnea [65, 66]. Severe respiratory distress occurs most often when the infant regurgitates, aspirates, and develops aspiration pneumonia. Infants with acute heroin withdrawal were found to have increased respiratory rates, leading to hypocapnia and an increase in blood alkalinity during the first week of life [67]. Glass found that the incidence of respiratory distress syndrome was actually decreased in NAS-affected infants, possibly because of chronic intrauterine stress, accelerated heroin-mediated maturation of lung function or perhaps both [67]. This decrease, however, is just one benefit among a long list of adverse effects resulting from intrauterine heroin exposure.

Autonomic nervous system – The signs seen during abstinence include sneezing, yawning, skin color changes (mottling), and water loss caused by increases in temperature and the shedding of tears. Behrendt and Green [68] found that approximately 40 percent of low-birth-weight infants born to heroin-dependent mothers had spontaneous generalized sweating. In comparison, this condition appeared in less than 1 percent of healthy low-birth-weight babies.

In an assessment of 135 newborns exposed in utero to heroin and/or methadone undergoing NAS, the following signs were seen in 50 percent or more of newborns: tremors (mild or marked and disturbed and undisturbed), high pitched cry, continuous high pitched cry, sneezing, increased muscle tone, frantic sucking of the fists, regurgitation, sleeps < 3 hours after feeding, respiratory rate > 60/minute, poor feeding, hyperactive Moro reflex, and loose stools [69].

## Assessment and Diagnosis

The level of fetal drug exposure can be affected by: the amount and purity of the drugs taken by the mother; the length of drug use and the mother's drug metabolism; and the individual kinetics of placental drug transfer. Because of these variables, it is difficult to clinically predict at birth whether a baby will develop NAS or, if developed, whether that NAS will be of a mild, moderate, or severe degree. As a result, careful assessment and diagnosis of newborns exposed to drugs in utero is the only way to determine if they will develop symptoms and warrant subsequent treatment. The use of a toxicology screening protocol at birth is helpful in monitoring for the onset of NAS. Urine or meconium toxicology screens are used. Meconium is the first intestinal discharge of the newborn infant. Consisting of epithelial cells, mucus, and bile, it also includes drugs the fetus was exposed to from about the 20th week of gestation [29].

## Assessment of NAS using a Scoring Tool

Not all drug-exposed newborns experience abstinence symptoms, therefore, routine prophylactic treatment is not recommended for NAS. Close observation of clinical signs is very important. The use of a severity score allows for the accurate evaluation of signs, avoids unnecessary treatment of mildly affected infants, and provides a methodology for the effective tapering of medications.

In the 1970s when NAS was being recognized and clinicians were considering treatment, no systematic, feasible, assessment, and treatment guideline was available for neonates. Scores to assess and treat abstinence in adults existed, i.e., the Himmelsbach Score [70], but those were not feasible for babies. With the undulating pattern of symptoms in the neonate vacillating from exacerbations of vigorous movements to sleep from exhaustion, a 24/7 assessment is appropriate. In the development of a score for newborns, the signs needed to be observed and categorized.

Signs of NAS are generally listed on score sheets according to the system that they affect: central nervous system, gastrointestinal system, respiratory system, and autonomic nervous system. It is important to confirm the diagnosis by maternal history, clinical findings of opioid use (e.g. track marks), urine toxicology screens, or meconium assessments. The laboratory assessments are confirmatory of exposure, but clinical examinations will determine if NAS appears. Scores permit administration of care systematically and selectively with avoidance of prolonged need for medication and hospital stay. A score allows for a "common language," decreased variability, and improves parent communication and involvement.

Assessment for other neonatal conditions with similar signs is important since the neonates are born to high risk women who generally have various morbidities. The following are conditions that can present with some of the signs similar to NAS which may have to be ruled out: septicemia, encephalitis, meningitis, postanoxic CNS irritation, hypoglycemia, hypocalcemia, and cerebral hemorrhage.

A number of scoring tools were developed during the 1970s–1990s and reported in the pediatric literature. The following scores have been published from 1975 to 2010: Neonatal Abstinence Score [15]; The Neonatal Drug Withdrawal Scoring System [16]; Ostrea Tool [71]; The Neonatal Narcotic Withdrawal Index [72]; Neonatal Withdrawal Inventory

**Finnegan Neonatal Abstinence Scoring Tool (FNAST)**

| Signs & Symptoms | Time | Score | AM | PM | Comments |
|---|---|---|---|---|---|
| **Central Nervous System Disturbances** | | | | | |
| Crying: Excessive High Pitched | | 2 | | | |
| Crying: Cont. High Pitched | | 3 | | | |
| Sleeps < 1 Hr After Feeding | | 3 | | | |
| Sleeps < 2 Hr After Feeding | | 2 | | | |
| Sleeps < 3 Hr After Feeding | | 1 | | | |
| Hyperactive Moro Reflex | | 2 | | | |
| Markedly Hyperactive Moro Reflex | | 3 | | | |
| Mild Tremors: Disturbed | | 1 | | | |
| Mod-Severe Tremors: Disturbed | | 2 | | | |
| Mild Tremors: Undisturbed | | 3 | | | |
| Mod-Severe Tremors: Undisturbed | | 4 | | | |
| Increased Muscle Tone | | 2 | | | |
| Excoriation (Specific Area) | | 1 | | | |
| Myoclonic Jerk | | 3 | | | |
| Generalized Convulsions | | 5 | | | |
| **Metabolic, Vasomotor And Respiratory Disturbance** | | | | | |
| Sweating | | 1 | | | |
| Fever < 101 (37.2–38.3c) | | 1 | | | |
| Fever > 101 (38.4c) | | 2 | | | |
| Frequent Yawning (> 3) | | 1 | | | |
| Mottling | | 1 | | | |
| Nasal Stuffiness | | 1 | | | |
| Sneezing (> 3) | | 1 | | | |
| Nasal Flaring | | 2 | | | |
| Respiratory Rate (> 60/Min) | | 1 | | | |
| Respiratory Rate (> 60/Min With Retractions) | | 2 | | | |
| **Gastrointestinal Disturbances** | | | | | |
| Excessive Sucking | | 1 | | | |
| Poor Feeding | | 2 | | | |
| Regurgitation | | 2 | | | |
| Projectile Vomiting | | 3 | | | |
| Loose Stools | | 2 | | | |
| Watery Stools | | 3 | | | |
| **Score** | | | | | |
| Total Score | | | | | |
| Average Daily Score | | | | | |
| Inter-Observer Reliability % | | | | | |
| Initials Of Scorer 1 | | | | | |
| Initials Of Scorer 2 | | | | | |

Patient ID:    Name:    Today's Weight:    DOB:    Date:

**Figure 14.1** The Finnegan Neonatal Abstinence Score

(NWI) [73]; MOTHER NAS Scale (modified Finnegan) [48]. All the scores except one use a dose of medication related to the weight (mg per kg per day divided into doses for the day). The MOTHER NAS Scale bases dose according to the score irrespective of weight.

The Finnegan Neonatal Abstinence Score is mentioned by the American Academy of Pediatrics in their guideline article for measuring the onset, progression and diminution of symptoms of abstinence [35] and is the most widely used tool in the United States today. The Lipsitz Neonatal Drug Withdrawal Scoring System [16] is used in some institutions but is not represented in the current literature. Use of the MOTHER NAS Scale is the standard instrument used in a number of clinical trials [74]. Figure 14.1 is a Finnegan scoring sheet.

The Neonatal Abstinence Score by Finnegan et al. [15] has an instructional manual and a DVD to train examiners to correctly administer the score. The manual assists with the following: accurately assesses opioid-exposed infants for the presence of abstinence signs; describes appropriate examination techniques required to evaluate NAS; reliability testing to achieve 90 percent reliability with other examiners in using the score. After orientation with this manual and DVD, an examiner can perform the score in 4–5 minutes. Since 1983, the score sheet has been translated into other languages [75].

## Nonpharmacological Interventions

Traditionally, comforting techniques such as swaddling, the use of a pacifier, and caregiving within a quiet, dimly lit environment have been recommended for reducing the signs of NAS. There is some clinical evidence to suggest that much NAS is really maternal abstinence syndrome, meaning separating babies from their primary caregivers causes distress. Treating babies in bright, noisy environments such as the NICU without maternal soothing has been anecdotally shown to worsen infant outcomes and increase the incidence of NAS. Such interventions are based on clinical experience rather than systematic evaluation and are primarily related to nursing care. This is not to say these techniques are not effective but to highlight a shift to a broader approach in which nonpharmacological measures focus on the importance of the mother and infant as an interactional dyad [76]. This has led to a number of studies that have identified breastfeeding as an important factor in decreasing NAS scores, the need for treatment, length of pharmacotherapy, and length of hospital stay in infants prenatally exposed to methadone or buprenorphine as important in decreasing [40, 77–79]. The act of breastfeeding is imbedded with behaviors that are soothing and comforting to the baby and promotes mother/infant attachment. This has led to a number of medical academies/societies, e.g. the Academy of Breastfeeding Medicine, 2015; the American Society of Addiction Medicine, 2012; and the World Health Organization 2014, to include in their Guideline recommendations that pregnant women maintained on methadone or buprenorphine who are not using illicit drugs, are engaged in treatment and are not HIV positive, be encouraged and supported in breastfeeding.

This same focus on the mother–infant dyad has led to integrating mothers as partners in care. A number of studies have examined the use of providing care within a rooming-in setting rather than in the usual NICU setting. Such an approach was first developed in Canada and received support through the Vermont Oxford Network (VON) NAS, a 3-year quality improvement project of 2013–15 [80]. Prior to the VON project, the majority of studies were conducted in Canada [81, 82], with 2 from England and Germany, respectively [83, 84]. A recent publication from the Dartmouth University hospital system that implemented a Plan-Do-Study-Act (PDSA) program in response to the VON project found that by providing extensive training on the NAS scoring tool, scoring the infant after on-demand feeding, using a standardized physician score interpretation, and keeping the infant in a rooming-in setting reduced the length of stay from 16.9 to 12.3 days and cumulative morphine dose from 13.7 to 6.6 mg [85].

The VON project also has led to studies examining the importance of standardizing hospital practices such as treatment protocols. Studies have found that utilizing a standard NAS treatment and weaning protocol for either morphine or methadone reduced duration of treatment and length of hospital stay [86], that staff education and the use of a standardized morphine protocol reduced length of stay [87], and that the use of explicit weaning guidelines resulted in shorter duration of treatment, length of stay, and lower rate of adjunctive drug therapy [88].

## Pharmacological Treatment

The need for and appropriate pharmacotherapy of neonatal opioid abstinence is based on the principles of accurate diagnosis and assessment. Since the signs of abstinence are nonspecific, the clinician must consider other serious neonatal conditions. In the neonatal period, pharmacotherapy is aimed at rapid clinical stabilization of the opioid-exposed infant followed by gradual reduction of the medication under careful medical supervision. Close assessment of the infant will ensure that mildly affected infants will not be treated unnecessarily and that infants who do require pharmacotherapy will not be allowed to develop severe abstinence with its attendant risk of significant morbidity and even mortality. For moderate to severely affected infants, medication dosage, in mg per kg, is related to the score and titrated up or down according to changes in scores. Medications are recommended when the score reaches a critical level and the neonate cannot be managed by supportive nursing measures. Dependent on a variety of factors, the average newborn will recover from NAS in 5–30 days and no untoward effects should occur as a result of this condition if appropriate assessment and treatment principles are provided.

The clinician should not procrastinate in providing medication for an infant whose NAS scores are at the treatment level. Waiting for severe symptoms to appear such as a seizure or dehydration is not warranted and precious time is lost in controlling the NAS. In the past, paregoric and tincture of opium were used to treat NAS. For a variety of reasons, not the least of which was the other substances within the medication (alcohol, anise oil, camphor, etc.) they are no longer prescribed. Diazepam and chlorpromazine are also not used because of their prolonged half-lives and associated complications [89].

Medications currently used by clinicians to treat NAS include: opioids (e.g. morphine, methadone, buprenorphine), anti-convulsants (e.g. phenobarbital), and centrally acting $\alpha_2$ agonists (e.g. clonidine). All of these medications have side effects and many include alcohol in the preparations. Morphine reduces bowel motility and loose stools in addition to facilitating feeding and interpersonal interaction. Morphine is also advantageous in that it has no alcohol and it has a short half-life. However, as with all opioids, it may cause apnea, sedation, hypotension, delayed gastric emptying, loss of bowel motility, and urinary retention.

It is generally assumed that opioid exposure precipitating NAS is best treated with another opioid; therefore, medications such as morphine and methadone have become the treatment of choice for NAS [35]. The recent recommendations by the American Academy of Pediatrics suggest carefully outlined regimens for orally administered methadone or morphine [35, 90]. Once the infant is clinically stabilized on a medication (based on decreasing abstinence scores), the total daily dosage can be lowered by 10 percent each day. When the medication is discontinued, the infant should be monitored in the hospital for rebound abstinence signs for at least 2 days [91, 92].

Kraft and colleagues conducted a series of open label randomized trials to examine the feasibility of using buprenorphine to treat NAS. The initial study compared sublingual buprenorphine versus a neonatal opium solution and found a nonsignificant reduction in length of treatment and duration of hospitalization in the buprenorphine group [93]. As this was the first study using buprenorphine to treat infants, a conservative dose was used. A subsequent study using an adjusted higher dose of buprenorphine found that the length of treatment was reduced by 40 percent ($p = 0.01$) and length of stay decreased by 24 percent ($p = 0.05$) for the buprenorphine treated infants compared to infants treated with morphine [94]. This group recently completed a double blind double dummy RCT comparing buprenorphine to morphine and found the duration of treatment to be significantly shorter with buprenorphine than methadone (15 days vs. 28 days, $p < 0.001$) [95].

Phenobarbital is frequently used as a second drug if morphine treatment does not adequately control the signs of abstinence, especially if exposure has been complicated by polydrug use [96, 97]. Phenobarbital is a nonspecific CNS depressant that offers the advantage of a broad spectrum of sedation controlling symptoms of irritability and insomnia in 50 percent of infants regardless of the mother's choice of drug. However, it does not control non-CNS signs such as loose stools; it depresses sucking; and, in larger doses, it can depress respirations and may mask the severity of NAS symptoms, thus infants need to be closely monitored for the possibility of over-sedation. But if physicians properly monitor the blood level of the phenobarbital, there should be no problem when using this medication for the treatment of NAS [98, 99]. Generally, phenobarbital is not recommended as the primary agent for treating NAS but as adjunct therapy in cases of polydrug exposure.

The Cochrane Controlled Trials Register [100, 101] examined the effectiveness and safety of opioid treatment compared to the use of sedatives and supportive care. In 285 infants meeting inclusion criteria in five studies, they concluded there is no evidence that phenobarbital (compared to supportive care alone) reduces treatment failure. In seven studies with 585 infants meeting inclusion criteria, they concluded that opioids (compared to supportive care alone) appeared to reduce both the time needed to regain birth weight and the duration of supportive care, but increased the duration of hospital stay. When compared to phenobarbital, opioids might reduce the incidence of seizures but there is no evidence of effect on treatment failure, further illustrating the superiority of opioids for the

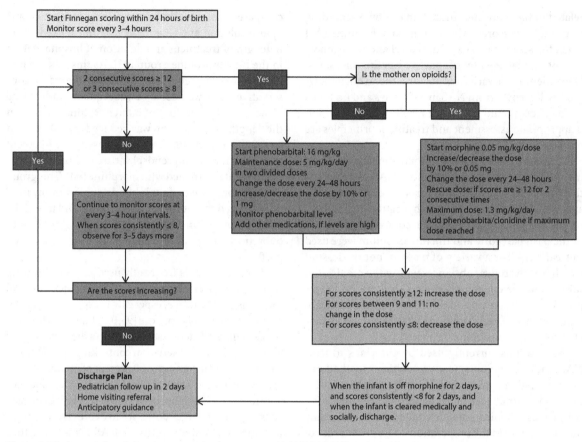

**Figure 14.2** A sample hospital management plan for neonates with NAS [102, 103]

treatment of NAS. An excellent review is found in an article by Kocherlakoda [102]. Figure 14.2 is a sample management plan based on this work.

Ebner and colleagues [104] compared the effects of phenobarbital and morphine hydrochloride and found that infants receiving morphine required a significantly shorter mean duration of treatment (9.9 days) than those treated with phenobarbital (17.7 days). They concluded that morphine is the preferable treatment for newborns with NAS.

Clonidine, an $\alpha_2$-adrenergic receptor agonist that can be used in combination with an opioid or other drug in older children and adults to reduce symptoms of autonomic over-activity such as rapid heart rate, hypertension, sweating, restlessness, and diarrhea has also been recommended by the American Academy of Pediatrics [35]. Experience with clonidine as a primary or a complementary treatment of NAS is limited [105, 106]. The theoretical risk of hypotension and bradycardia may always prohibit increasing its dose.

Bada and colleagues [107] studied whether clonidine treatment of NAS would result in a better neurobehavioral performance compared with morphine. Treatment duration was significantly longer for morphine and neurobehavioral scores (NNNS) improved significantly with clonidine but not with morphine. Clonidine-treated babies had lower height of arousal and excitability. The researchers concluded that clonidine may be a favorable alternative to morphine as a single-drug therapy for NAS. Evidence remains limited, with only one randomized, controlled trial conducted and no long-term studies available. Larger, prospective, multicenter randomized trials are warranted to assess the efficacy and safety of clonidine in the treatment of NAS.

Because of its potential for precipitating severe abstinence symptoms, naloxone should not be given to newborns exposed to opioids in utero although it is occasionally given to newborns having breathing problems to reverse the acquired effects of pain medications typically administered to the mother during labor and delivery.

Concern is often voiced regarding the developmental outcome of infants undergoing NAS. Albeit, the available data is limited, it does not support an association with severity of NAS (i.e. NAS requiring pharmacological treatment vs. moderate to mild NAS) with long-term developmental outcome [108]. In addition, studies on long-term developmental outcome of children prenatally exposed to opioids have not found consistent evidence of adverse outcomes with negative findings usually confounded by the environment [109].

Disclosure: The author (LF) discloses that the aforementioned instructional manual and DVD are copyrighted and that she receives royalties from their sales.

# References

1. Heroin Timeline. Heroin addiction. Available at: www.heroinaddiction.com/heroin_timeline.html. Accessed October 12, 2013.

2. Merry J. A social history of heroin addiction. *Br J Addict Alcohol Other Drugs* 1975; 70(3):307–10.

3. Courtwright D. *Dark Paradise: Opiate Addiction in America Before 1940*. Cambridge, MA: Harvard University Press; 1982.

4. Menninger-Lerchenthal E. Die morphin kranheit der neugeborenen morphine stischer mutter Monatsschr. *F Kinderh* 1934; 60:182–93.

5. Happel T. J. Morphinism in its relation to the sexual functions and appetite and its effects on the offspring of the users of the drug. *Tr M Soc Tennessee* 1892; 162–79.

6. Earle F. B. Maternal opium habit and infant mortality. *Med Standard (Chicago)* 1888; 3:2.

7. OD. Fetal morphine addiction, queries and minor notes. *JAMA* 1903; 40:1092.

8. Perlstein M. A. Congenital morphinism: A rare cause of convulsions in the newborn. *J Am Med Assoc* 1947;135(10):633.

9. Goodfriend M. J., Shey I. A., Klein M. D. The effects of maternal narcotic addiction on the newborn. *Am J Obstet Gynecol* 1956; 71(1):29–36.

10. Cobrinik R. W., Hood R. T. Jr, Chusid E. The effect of maternal narcotic addiction on the newborn infant; review of literature and report of 22 cases. *Pediatrics* 1959; 24(2):288–304.

11. National Consensus Development Panel on Effective Medical Treatment of Opiate Addiction. Effective medical treatment of opiate addiction. *JAMA* 1998; 280(22):1936–43.

12. Reddy A. M., Harper R. G., Stern G. Observations on heroin and methadone withdrawal in the newborn. *Pediatrics* 1971; 48(3):353–8.

13. Blinick G., Jerez E., Wallach R. C. Methadone maintenance, pregnancy, and progeny. *J Am Med Assoc* 1973; 225:477–9.

14. Zelson C., Rubio E., Wasserman E. Neonatal narcotic addiction: 10-year observation. *Pediatrics* 1971; 48:178.

15. Finnegan L. P., Kron R. E., Connoughton J. F., Emich J. P. A Scoring System for Evaluation and Treatment of the Neonatal Abstinence Syndrome: A New Clinical and Research Tool. In P. I. Morselli, F. Sereni, editors. *Basic and Therapeutic Aspects of Perinatal Pharmacology*. New York: Raven Press; 1975, pp. 139–53.

16. Lipsitz P. J. A proposed narcotic withdrawal score for use with newborn infants. *Clin Pediatr* 1975; 14(6):592–4.

17. Auriacombe M., Fatséas M., Dubernet J., Daulouède J. P., Tignol J. French field experience with buprenorphine. *Am J Addict* 2004; 13(suppl 1): S17–S28.

18. Center for Substance Abuse Treatment. *Clinical Guidelines for the Use of Buprenorphine in the Treatment of Opioid Addiction. Treatment Improvement Protocol (TIP) Series 40*. Rockville, MD: Substance Abuse and Mental Health Administration; 2004. DHHS publication (SMA) 04-3939.

19. Marquet P., Chevrel J., Lavignasse P., Merle L., Lachâtre G. Buprenorphine withdrawal syndrome in a newborn. *Clin Pharmacol Ther* 1997; 62(5): 569–71.

20. Kayemba-Kay's S., Laclyde J. P. Buprenorphine withdrawal syndrome in newborns: A report of 13 cases. *Addiction* 2003; 98(11):1599–604.

21. Rao R., Desai N. S. Oxycontin and neonatal abstinence syndrome. *J Perinatol*. 2002; 22(4):324–5.

22. Jansson L. M. Neonatal abstinence syndrome. www.uptodate.com. Accessed December 16.

23. McCarthy J. J., Leamon M. H., Willits N. H., Salo R. The effects of methadone dose regimen on neonatal abstinence syndrome. *J Addict Med* 2015; 9:105–10.

24. Kaltenbach K., Jones H. J. Neonatal abstinence syndrome: Presentation and treatment considerations. *J Addict Med* 2016; 10(4):217–33.

25. Patrick S. W., Schumacher R. E., Bennyworth B. D., et al. Neonatal abstinence syndrome and associated health care expenditures. *JAMA* 2012; 307(18): 1934–40.

26. Ko J. Y., Patrick S. W., Tong V. T., et al. Incidence of neonatal abstinence syndrome – 28 states, 1999–2013. *MMWR* 2016; 65(31):799–802.

27. Patrick S. W., Davis M. M., Lehmann C. U., Cooper W. O. Increasing incidence and geographical distribution of neonatal abstinence syndrome: United States 2009–2012. *J Perinatol* 2015; 35:650–5.

28. Vallapiano N. L. G., Winkleman T. N. A., Kozhimannil K. B., Davis M. M., Patrick S. W. Rural and urban differences in neonatal abstinence syndrome and maternal opioid use, 2004–2013. *JAMA Pediatr* 2016; doi: 10.1001/jamapediatrics.2016.3750.

29. Finnegan L. P., Kandall S. R. Neonatal abstinence syndromes. In J. Aranda, S. J. Jaffe, editors. *Neonatal and Pediatric Pharmacology: Therapeutic Principles in Practice*. 3rd ed. Philadelphia: Lippincott Williams & Wilkins; 2005.

30. Gillogley K. M., Evans A. T., Hansen R. L., Samuels S. J., Batra K. K. The perinatal impact of cocaine, amphetamine, and opiate use detected by universal intrapartum screening. *Am J Obstet Gynecol* 1990; 163:1535–42.

31. Connaughton J. F., Reeser D., Schut J., Finnegan L. P. Perinatal addiction: Outcome and management. *Am J Obstet Gynecol* 1977; 129:679–86.

32. Rorke L. B., Reeser D. S., Finnegan L. P. Nervous system lesions in infants of opiate dependent mothers. *Pediatr Res* 1977; 11:565.

33. Holbrook A. M., Baxter J. K., Jones H. E., et al. Infections and obstetrical outcomes in opioid-dependent pregnant women maintained on methadone or buprenorphine. *Addiction* 2012; 107(Suppl. 1):83–90.

34. Finnegan L. P., Hagan T., Kaltenbach K. Opioid dependence: Scientific foundations for clinical practice, pregnancy and substance abuse: Perspectives and directions. *Bull N Y Acad Med* 1991; 67(3):223–9.

35. Hudak M. L., Tan R. C. Committee on drugs; committee on fetus and newborn American academy of pediatrics clinical report. Neonatal drug withdrawal. *Pediatrics* 2012; 129(2):e540–60.

36. Kaltenbach K., Holbrook A., Coyle M., et al. Predicting treatment for neonatal abstinence syndrome in infants born to women maintained on opioid agonist medication. *Addiction* 2012; 107 (Suppl. 1):45–52.

37. Jansson L. M., Diepietro J. A., Elko A., Velez M. Infant autonomic functioning and neonatal abstinence. *Drug Alcohol Depend* 2010; 109:198–204.

38. Seligman N. S., Salva N., Hayes E. J., et al. Predicting length of treatment for neonatal abstinence syndrome in methadone exposed infants. *Am J Obstet Gynecol* 2008; 396:e1–7.

39. Dryden C., Young D., Hepburn M., Mactier H. Maternal methadone use in pregnancy: Factors associated with the development of neonatal abstinence syndrome and implications for healthcare resources. *Br J Obstet Gynecol* 2009; 116(5):665–71.

40. Wachman E. M., Newby P. K., Vreeland J., et al. The relationship between maternal opioid agonists and psychiatric medications on length of hospitalization for neonatal abstinence. *J Addict Med* 2011; 5(4): 293–9.

41. Pritham U. A., Paul J. A., Hayes M. J. Opioid dependency in pregnancy and length of stay for neonatal abstinence syndrome. *J Obstet Gynecol Neonatal Nurs* 2012; 41(20):180–90.

42. Choo R. E., Huestis M. A., Schroeder J. R., Shin A. S., Jones H. E. Neonatal abstinence syndrome in methadone-exposed infants is altered by level of prenatal tobacco exposure. *Drug Alcohol Depend* 2004; 75:253–60.

43. Jones H. E., Heil S. H., Tuten M., et al. Cigarette smoking in opioid dependent pregnant women: Neonatal and maternal outcomes. *Drug Alcohol Depend* 2013; 131(3):271–7.

44. Gibson K. S., Starks S., Kumar D., Bailit J. L. Relationship between gestational age and the severity of neonatal abstinence syndrome. *Addiction* 2017; 112(4):711–6.

45. Doberczak T. M., Kandall S. R., Wilets I. Neonatal opiate abstinence syndrome in term and preterm infants. *J Pediatr* 1991; 118:933–7.

46. Ruwanpathirana R., Abedel-Latif M. E., Burns L., et al. Prematurity reduces the severity and need for treatment of neonatal abstinence syndrome. *Acta Paediatr* 2015; 104:e188–e94.

47. Dysart K., Hsieh H., Kaltenbach K., Greenspan J. S. Sequela of preterm versus term infants born to mothers on a methadone maintenance program: Differential course of neonatal abstinence syndrome. *J Perinat Med* 2007; 35:344–6.

48. Jones H. E., Kaltenbach K., Heil S. H., et al., Neonatal abstinence syndrome after methadone or buprenorphine exposure. *NEJM* 2010; 363:2320–31.

49. Gaalema D. E., Scott T. L., Heil S. H., et al. Differences in the profile of neonatal abstinence syndrome signs in methadone versus buprenorphine-exposed infants. *Addiction* 2012; 107(Suppl.):53–62.

50. Unger A., Jagsch R., Bawert A., et al. Are male neonates more vulnerable to neonatal abstinence syndrome than female neonates? *Gender Medicine* 2011; 8(6):355–64.

51. Holbrook A., Kaltenbach K. Gender and NAS: Does sex matter? *Drug Alcohol Depend* 2010; 112(1–2): 156–9.

52. Wachman E. M., Hayes M. J., Brown M. S., et al. Association of OPRM1 and COMT single-nucleotide polymorphisms with hospital length of stay and

treatment of neonatal abstinence syndrome. *JAMA* 2013; 309(17):1821–7.

53. Wachman E. M., Hayes M. J., Lester B. M., et al. Epigenetic variation in the mu-opioid receptor gene in infants with neonatal abstinence syndrome. *J Pediatr* 2014; 165(3):472–8.

54. Wachman E. M., Hayes M. J., Sherva R., et al. Variations in opioid receptor genes in neonatal abstinence syndrome. *Drug Alcohol Depend* 2015; 155:253–9.

55. Cleary B. J., Donelly J., Strawbridge J., et al. Methadone dose and neonatal abstinence syndrome – Systematic review and meta-analysis. *Addiction* 2010; 105:2071–84.

56. Jones H. E., Jansson L. M., O'Grady K. E., Kaltenbach K. The relationship between maternal methadone dose at delivery and neonatal outcomes: Methodological and design considerations. *Neurotoxicol Teratol* 2013; 39:110–5.

57. Jones H. E., Dengler E., Garrison A., et al. Neonatal outcomes and their relationship to buprenorphine dose during pregnancy. *Drug Alcohol Depend* 2014; 134:414–47.

58. Brogly S. B., Saia K. A., Walley A. Y., Du H. M., Sebastian P. Prenatal buprenorphine versus methadone exposure and neonatal abstinence syndrome: Systematic review and meta-analysis. *Am J Epidemiol* 2014; 180:673–86.

59. Jones H. E., Finnegan L. P., Kaltenbach K. Methadone and buprenorphine for the management of opioid dependence in pregnancy. *Drugs* 2012; 72(6):747–57.

60. Finnegan L. P. Neonatal abstinence syndrome: Assessment and pharmacotherapy. In F. F. Rubaltelli, B. Granati, editors. *Neonatal Therapy: An Update*. New York: Elsevier; 1986, pp. 122–46.

61. Kron R. E., Litt M., Phoenix M. D., Finnegan L. P. Neonatal narcotic abstinence: Effects of pharmacotherapeutic agents and maternal drug usage on nutritive sucking behavior. *J Pediatr* 1976; 88: 637–41.

62. Herzlinger R. A., Kandall S. R., Vaughan H. G. Neonatal seizures associated with narcotic withdrawal. *J Pediatr* 1977; 91:638–41.

63. Kandall S. R., Doberczak T. M., Mauer K. R., Strashun R. H., Korts D. C. Opiate v CNS depressant therapy in neonatal drug abstinence syndrome. *Am J Dis Child* 1983; 137:378–82.

64. Weinberger S. M., Kandall S. R., Doberczak T. M., Thornton J. C., Bernstein J. Early weight-change patterns in neonatal abstinence. *Am J Dis Child* 1986; 140:829–32.

65. Finnegan L. P. Pulmonary problems encountered by the infant of the drug-dependent mother. *Clin Chest Med* 1980; 1:311–25.

66. Finnegan L.P. Influence of maternal drug dependence on the newborn. In S. Kacew, S. Lock, editors. *Toxicologic and Pharmacologic Principles in Pediatrics*. Washington, DC: Hemisphere; 1988.

67. Glass L., Rajegowda B. K., Kahn E. J., Floyd M. V. Effect of heroin on respiratory rate and acid–base status in the newborn. *N Engl J Med* 1972; 286:746–8.

68. Behrendt H., Green M. Nature of the sweating deficit of prematurely born neonates. *N Engl J Med* 1972; 286:1376–9.

69. NIDA Services Research Monograph Series. Drug Dependence in Pregnancy: Clinical Management of Mother and Child, Loretta Finnegan, Ed. ADAMHA, 1979.

70. Himmelsbach C. K. The morphine abstinence syndrome, its nature and treatment. *Ann Intern Med* 1941; 15:829–39.

71. Ostrea E. M., Chavez C. J., Strauss M. E. A study of factors that influence the severity of neonatal narcotic withdrawal. *J Pediatr* 1976; 88:642–5.

72. Green M., Suffet F. The neonatal narcotic withdrawal index: A device for the improvement of care in the abstinence syndrome. *Am J Drug Alcohol Abuse* 1981; 8(2):203–13.

73. Zahordony W., Rom C., Whitney W., et al. The neonatal withdrawal inventory: A simplified score of newborn withdrawal. *Dev Behav Pediatr* 1998; 19(2):89–93.

74. Kraft W. K., van den Anker J. N. Pharmacologic management of the opioid neonatal abstinence syndrome. *Pediatr Clin N Am* 2012; 59:1147–65.

75. D'Apolito K., Finnegan L. Assessing Signs & Symptoms of Neonatal Abstinence Using the Finnegan Scoring Tool, An Inter-Observer Reliability Program, Neo Advances, 2010. www.neoadvances.com

76. Velez M., Jansson L. M. The opioid dependent mother and newborn dyad: Non-pharmacological care. *J Addict Med* 2008; 2(3):133–20.

77. Wachman E. M., Newby P. K., Vreeland J., et al. The relationship between maternal opioid agonists and psychiatric medications on length of hospitalization for neonatal abstinence. *J Addict Med* 2011; 5(4): 293–9.

78. Welle-Strand G. K., Skurtveit S., Jansson L. M. Breastfeeding reduces the need for withdrawal treatment in opioid-exposed infants. *Acta Paediatr* 2014; 165(3):440–6.

79. Short V., Gannon M., Abatemarco D. J. Association between breastfeeding and length of stay among infants diagnosed with NAS: A population based study of in-hospital births. *Breastfeed* 2016; 11:343–9.

80. Vermont Oxford Network (VON) www.public .vtoxford.org

81. Abrahams R. R., Key S. A., Payne S., et al. Rooming-in compared with standard care for newborns of mothers using methadone or heroin. *Can Fam Physicians* 2007; 53(10):1722–30.

82. Newman A., Davies G. A., Dow K., et al. Rooming-in care for infants of opioid dependent mothers: Implementation and evaluation at a tertiary care hospital. *Can Fam Physicians* 2012; 61(12):555–61.

83. Saiki T., Lee S., Hannam S. Neonatal abstinence syndrome – Postnatal ward versus neonatal unit management. *Eur J Pediatr* 2010; 169:95–8.

84. Hunseler C., Bruckle M., Roth B., Kribs A. Neonatal opiate withdrawal and rooming-in: A retrospective analysis of a single study experiment. *Klin Pediatri* 2013; 225(5):247–51.

85. Holmes A. V., Atwood E. C., Whalen B., et al. Rooming-in to treat neonatal abstinence syndrome: Improved family centered care and lower cost. *Pediatrics*, 2016; doi: 10.1542/peds.2015-2929.

86. Hall E. S., Wexelblatt S. L., Crowley M., et al. A multicenter cohort study of treatments and hospital outcomes in neonatal abstinence syndrome. *Pediatrics*, 2014; 14(2):e527–e34.

87. Asti L., Magers J. S., Keels E., Wispe J., McClead R. E. A quality improvement project to reduce length of stay for neonatal abstinence syndrome. *Pediatrics*, 2015; 135(6):e1494–1500.

88. Hall E. S., Wexelblatt S. L., Crowley M. Implementation of a neonatal abstinence syndrome scoring weaning protocol. *Pediatrics*, 2015; 136(4):e803–10.

89. Osborn D. A., Jeffery H. E., Cole M. J. Sedatives for opiate withdrawal in newborn infants. *Cochrane Database Syst Rev* 2010; (10): Art. No. CD002053; doi: 10.1002/14651858.CD002053.pub3.

90. Jackson L., Ting A., McKay S., Galea P., Skeoch C. A randomized controlled trial of morphine versus phenobarbitone for neonatal abstinence syndrome. *Arch Dis Child* 2004; 89(4 Special Issue):F300–4.

91. Finnegan L. P., Kaltenbach K. Neonatal abstinence syndrome. In R. A. Hoekelman, S. B. Friedman, N. Nelson, editors. *Primary Pediatric Care*. 2nd ed. St. Louis, MO: CV Mosby; 1992, pp. 1367–8.

92. Kandall S. R. Treatment strategies for drug-exposed neonates. *Clin Perinatol* 1999; 26:231–43.

93. Kraft W. K., Gibson E., Dysart K., et al. Sublingual buprenorphine for treatment of neonatal abstinence syndrome: A randomized trial. *Pediatrics* 2008; 122(3):e601–7.

94. Kraft W. K., Dysart K., Greenspan J. S. Revised dose schema of sublingual buprenorphine in the treatment of neonatal opioid syndrome. *Addiction* 2011; 106(3):574–80.

95. Kraft W. K., Adeniyi-Jones S. C., Chervoneva I., et al. Buprenorphine for the treatment of the neonatal abstinence syndrome. *N Engl J Med* 2017; doi: 10.1065/NEJMoa1614835.

96. Sarkar S., Dunn S. M. Management of neonatal abstinence syndrome in neonatal intensive care units: A national survey. *J Perinatol* 2006;26(1):15–7.

97. O'Grady M. J., Hopewell J., White M. J. Management of neonatal abstinence syndrome: A national survey and review of practice. *Arch Dis Child Fetal Neonatal Ed* 2009; 94(4):F249–52.

98. Weiner S. M., Finnegan L. P. Drug withdrawal in the neonate. In Carter B., Gardner S., editors. *Handbook of Neonatal Intensive Care*, 8th ed. St. Louis, MO: Mosby-Year Book Inc; 2016.

99. Bio L. L., Siu A., Poon C. Y. Update on the pharmacologic management of neonatal abstinence syndrome. *J Perinatol* 2011; 31(11):692–701.

100. Osborn D. A., Jeffery H. E., Cole M. Sedatives for opiate withdrawal in newborn infants. *Cochrane Database Syst Rev* 2002; (3):CD002053.

101. Osborn D. A., Jeffery H. E., Cole M. Opiate treatment for opiate withdrawal in newborn infants. *Cochrane Database Syst Rev* 2005; (3):CD002059.

102. Kocherlakota P., Neonatal abstinence syndrome, *Pediatrics* 2014 Aug; 134(2):e547–61.

103. North Carolina Pregnancy & Opioids Exposure Project. www.ncpoep.org/guidance-document/neonatal-abstinence-syndrome-overview/appendix-a-neonatal-abstinence-syndrome-nas-scoring-explanation/

104. Ebner N., Rohrmeister K., Winklbaur B., et al. Management of neonatal abstinence syndrome in neonates born to opioid maintained women. *Drug Alcohol Depend* 2007;87(2–3):131–8.

105. Leikin J. B., Mackendrick W. P., Maloney G. E., et al. Use of clonidine in the prevention and management of neonatal abstinence syndrome. *Clin Toxicol (Phila)* 2009; 47(6):551–5.

106. Esmaeili A., Keinhorst A. K., Scuster T., et al. Treatment of neonatal abstinence syndrome with clonidine and chloral hydrate. *Acta Paediatr* 2010; 99(2):209–14.

107. Bada H. S., Sithisarn T., Gibson J., et al. Morphine versus clonidine for neonatal abstinence syndrome. *Pediatrics* 2015 Feb; 135(2):e383–91.

108. Kaltenbach K., Finnegan L. P. Neonatal abstinence: Pharmacotherapy and developmental outcome. *Neurobehav Toxicol Teratol* 1986; 8:353–5.

109. Behnke M., Smith V. C. Prenatal substance abuse: Short and long term effects of the exposed fetus. *Pediatrics* 2013; 131:e1009–e24.

# Chapter 5

# Breastfeeding and the Substance-Exposed Dyad

Lauren M. Jansson and Stephen W. Patrick

## Introduction

The problems associated with maternal substance use disorders (SUDs) and effects on the infant and child have expanded in the United States in the past two decades without precedent [1, 2]. Optimal care of the substance-exposed dyad is multidimensional, and breastfeeding is one strategy that can benefit both mother and baby. Breastmilk is optimal nutrition for the newborn, and it confers well-known short- and long-term health and developmental benefits for the infant. For a population of infants at elevated risk for medical, developmental, and emotional-behavioral concerns, this benefit stands to be substantial. Additionally, breastfed opioid-exposed infants have less severe neonatal abstinence syndrome (NAS) as compared to formula-fed infants [3]. Breastfeeding confers similarly positive benefits for the mother, including health and self-regulatory benefits, improved attachment and communication with the infant, improved functioning via stress reduction, enhanced self-concept as a caregiver [4] and increased sensitivity to infant cues [5]. Women with a history of SUD are a population of women at particular risk for medical concerns, poor dyadic communication patterns, deficits in parental functioning and poor self-regulation; breastfeeding promotion, applied to appropriate dyads, could be a cost-effective mechanism to improve the physical and psychological trajectory of substance-exposed dyads [6]. Yet, despite the particularly salient benefits of lactation, breastfeeding rates in this expanding population are low, approximately 24 percent as compared to 79 percent of the general population [7, 8]. Reasons for these low rates of lactation are myriad, and can result from the mother, the infant, the dyad, the provider/institution/environment and shifting combinations of all.

## Understanding and Treating the Lactating Mother with a Substance Use Disorder (SUD)

### SUD and Lactation

The new mother with an SUD frequently presents with multiple challenges which can interfere with the initiation and continuation of breastfeeding. Idiosyncratic cultural norms among women with SUD may affect their decision to breastfeed. Multigenerational addiction, poor role models for lactation, or few peers breastfeeding their infants may have mothers seldom considering breastfeeding as a viable option. Breastfed newborns feed more frequently than formula-fed newborns and require maternal attention almost exclusively, and therefore provide more frequent cueing for maternal attention. Mothers with SUDs can find normally rewarding infant cues as stressful, and heightened levels of stress in a low reward environment increases craving for substances of abuse that will, by experience, bring relief from stress. Thus, the act of caring for an infant may be a trigger for relapse to substance use [9]; this risk may be heightened in breastfed infants. On the other hand, teaching relapse prevention skills and promoting breastfeeding concurrently can positively affect both behaviors, at least as related to cigarette smoking [10]. Hallmarks of SUDs which can result from or precede chronic use of drugs, such as increased impulsivity and risk taking, poor attention, emotional dysregulation, and poor self-regulation may all impair the mother's ability to initiate and sustain breastfeeding, and may additionally have implications for the safety of lactation. Individuals with SUDs frequently have low tolerance for pain or setbacks, putting them at risk for increased stress and consequent relapse to substance use. (i.e. "what if breastfeeding hurts/the baby fails to latch/doesn't get enough milk/rejects my breast (i.e. me)"?) Other fears may include lack of family support for lactation, and the fear of passage of medications used to treat opioid use disorders or other substances taken by the mother into breastmilk. These fears should be addressed in counseling both prior to and after birth.

## Active Maternal Addiction and Lactation

Ideally, the woman with an SUD who desires lactation is abstinent from substance use, stable on medication-assisted treatment for an opioid use disorder (if warranted) and in a comprehensive SUD treatment program, but this is not always the scenario that presents at the time of delivery. It cannot be presumed that women who desire lactation are abstinent from substance use/misuse as there is evidence that women who are in active addiction patterns do choose to breastfeed their infants [11]. Lactation is contraindicated in women with active addiction patterns regardless of substance (including marijuana); however, the determination of active addiction vs. stable recovery is not always readily definable, particularly for a provider who is not familiar with addictions or the mother's history, and reliance on biologic screening tests and maternal history can be problematic. Further, even women that are stable in their recovery are at heightened risk for relapse in the postpartum period [12], not infrequently due to the guilt associated with observing their infant experience NAS, thus care providers should focus on relapse prevention.

Maternal active addiction can result in somnolence, altered sensoriums and/or responses to the infant and a chaotic or violent environment, all of which can portend risk to the infant's development over the long term and their safety in the short term, and a more specific risk to the breastfed infant who must necessarily be in proximity to his mother. The breastfed infant may be at increased risk for smothering due to poor positioning while breastfeeding, or exposure to substances in breastmilk or via secondary exposures, which can be significant [13]. Additionally, active addiction patterns often include drug seeking/taking activities that may place the woman and her infant in risky situations, including prostitution, unsafe locations, and potentially violent or chaotic environments.

All potential substances of misuse are transmitted into breastmilk and to the infant, and some have been documented to provide significant morbidity to the breastfeeding infant. Since most women with SUD are polysubstance using, a discussion of individual substance effects is somewhat artificial. Additionally, there is a dearth of information on individual substances in breastmilk, and that is likely to remain the case, since this research is ethically difficult to perform. However, a synopsis is included here for completeness' sake:

Cocaine appears variably in breastmilk, and high concentrations are possible [14]; exposure has resulted in infant intoxication [15]. Amphetamines frequently contain adulterants, may appear in breastmilk days after use [16, 17], are found in concentrations 2.8–7.5 times plasma concentrations, and can cause irritability and death [18]. PCP can be highly concentrated in breastmilk [19]. Alcohol can produce alterations in sleep cycles [20] and infant development [21]. Benzodiazepines, when prescribed, are likely to present minimal risk to the breastfed infant, but drug-drug interactions may increase the risk for CNS depression [22]. Irritability, lethargy, poor weight gain and apnea have been reported [23]. Opioids such as oxycodone can cause CNS depression in 20 percent of infants [24] and codeine may cause a dose dependent CNS depression, particularly in ultrarapid metabolizers to morphine [24]; one death has been reported [25]. Because of these risks among ultrarapid metabolizers, the US Food and Drug Administration recommends that breastfeeding women not be prescribed codeine or tramadol [26]. Research on marijuana use and breastfeeding is several decades old, and marijuana today is approximately four times as potent as it was in most of these earlier studies [27]. Marijuana delivered via breastmilk is absorbed and metabolized by the infant [28], may affect the ontogeny of various neurotransmitter systems, leading to changes in neurobiologic functioning [29], can cause sedation, weakness and poor feeding [30], significant health and other effects making it a potentially dangerous exposure via breastmilk [31]. Women should be counseled that breastfeeding is not recommended with marijuana use, and that continued use of substances that can cause harm (even if legal) throughout pregnancy is strongly suggestive of having a substance use disorder.

## Medical Conditions, Psychiatric Conditions, Medications and Lactation

Women with SUDs more often than not present with medical or psychiatric co-morbidities, which may deter the choice of lactation, rightfully or not. Concurrent HIV infection is a contraindication to lactation, but other infections, such as hepatitis B/C, not necessarily contraindications to lactation (hepatitis C is a contraindication if bleeding or cracked nipples present), or smoking cigarettes may deter women from breastfeeding due to lack of information or fears of compounding other exposures. Co-promotion of smoking cessation/relapse prevention and breastfeeding has shown benefit in these patients [10]. Maternal psychiatric concerns in this population, most commonly depression and anxiety [32], can deter a mother from breastfeeding in several ways. These disorders can affect a mother's self-confidence as a caregiver, her ability to read infant cues of hunger/satiation, her capacity for seeing her damaged self/body as "safe" to provide nutrition for her infant or her self-efficacy to advocate for lactation for herself and her infant. Psychiatric co-morbidities are often treated with medications during the perinatal period, as untreated maternal psychiatric illness may be harmful to both mother and infant. Medications used to treat these conditions are all transferred into human milk; most are compatible with breastfeeding, with some exceptions (i.e. Haldol), but these too may deter women from breastfeeding for fear of infant exposure via breastmilk compounding other prenatal and postnatal exposures. Medications used to treat maternal opioid use disorders during pregnancy and postpartum (i.e. methadone and buprenorphine) are transmitted into breastmilk in low concentrations and are not contraindications to lactation [33, 34]. However, mothers who need to access treatment programs daily to obtain these medications that do not accept the presence of the infant may find logistical barriers that hinder their ability to breastfeed the infant.

## Maternal Sexual Trauma and Lactation

Physical, emotional, and sexual abuse are common in women with SUD, in both past histories and current pregnancy [35]. Histories of sexual abuse are frequently unrecognized, and can be a major factor in the inability for some women to consider or sustain lactation. Women with histories of sexual abuse often feel shame or self-blame for issues surrounding nudity, breasts, childbirth, or sensations related to breastfeeding an infant. Expressions including "my body in the baby's mouth is disgusting," or "breastfeeding is perverted" are common. Poor self-esteem or self-efficacy in women who have experienced sexual trauma often

results in early cessation of breastfeeding. Women may feel mistrust or hostility related to the infant's need for her body, particularly for older infants who may play at the breast, or infants demanding nighttime feedings. Psychiatric co-morbidities are common in women who have experienced sexual trauma, and range from depression to PTSD. The act of breastfeeding an infant combined with the process of childbirth may predispose this group of women to flashbacks, especially in the perinatal period, when strangers (i.e. medical staff, particularly men) have the need to expose and touch her body. Many women who have experienced violence can only give the infant pumped breastmilk, as the feeling or viewing of an infant suckling is intolerable, as is "forced" exposure of the body. Women who have been victims of sexual violence may experience pain out of proportion to clinical findings, and the pain associated with breastfeeding initiation can be a trigger for depression or PTSD [36]. Sleep disorders are common among sexual assault survivors which can increase risk for depression, but the risk for these is lowered in breastfeeding as opposed to formula feeding mothers [37].

## Treating the Lactating Mother with an SUD

Despite these challenges, many women with an SUD are willing to breastfeed and thus should be encouraged to do so. The only two absolute contraindications to breastfeeding in the United States are active substance use and HIV positivity. Ideally, the mother with an SUD who presents desiring to breastfeed her infant has been identified during the course of her prenatal care, and preparation for breastfeeding can be done. Issues related to trauma exposure, psychiatric co-morbidities and feelings that commonly arise when seeing the infant experience NAS at the breast can be preemptively addressed. Lactation support can be very helpful in the hospital and outpatient clinic to promote the maternal–infant dyad and address difficulties. By using trauma-informed and trauma-responsive care, the lactation support can address issues with previous abuse and use breastfeeding as relapse prevention. Available maternal treatment histories of active use and sobriety periods can be used to determine appropriate candidates for breastfeeding.

For women who lack prenatal care and in whom a thorough history is not known, a thorough assessment of the mother is warranted, to include: personal and drug use history, engagement (or not) in treatment for SUD,

129

psychiatric co-morbidities, treatment (or not) and medication used to treat psychiatric co-morbidities, medical history and medications, violence/trauma exposure, family and community supports and plans for postpartum and SUD treatment and pediatric care.

When considering psychiatric medications and lactation, a multidisciplinary approach involving primary care, obstetric, psychiatric, and pediatric providers is warranted, as is using the safest effective medication (i.e. short as opposed to long-acting), carefully evaluating risk and benefits, and assuring careful and experienced monitoring of the infant. However, women who are stable on a specific psychiatric medication should not be switched to one with a shorter half-life solely for breastfeeding, as switching medication can increase relapse risk. Stable women on medication-assisted treatment with methadone or buprenorphine as part of SUD treatment who are candidates for lactation should be encouraged to do so regardless of dose. There is evidence that buprenorphine concentrations in breastmilk are dose-dependent [34], but buprenorphine is not substantially absorbed orally. Buprenorphine and metabolite concentrations in infants of buprenorphine maintained women at 2 weeks of age are low or nondetectable [34]. Women are often under the misconception that she is "treating" the NAS by providing buprenorphine or methadone in breast milk. Gentle disabusing of this misconception can be helpful so that women remain on the most effective dose, without worrying about the infant's treatment.

Maternal somnolence in the postpartum period is not uncommon. Somnolence can be related to guilt and depression, the demands of the newborn, significant other, family and social services interventions or pressures or sleep disorders, which are common in women with SUDs. The dose of methadone for those women in maintenance therapy often requires a downward adjustment after delivery due to diminished volumes of distribution for the medication. For women with trauma histories, an evaluation for depression, guilt and issues surrounding victimization is necessary. For this population of women, revictimization is not uncommon and should be assessed. Feeding the infant only pumped breastmilk may be a red flag for sexual trauma, which if discovered during the postpartum period has implications for the sustainability of lactation and should be addressed by appropriate professionals. Women should never be forced to breastfeed or be made to feel guilty if they cannot or chose not to breastfeed.

Maternal education is an important component of successful lactation, and ideally this begins in the prenatal period. Teaching regarding NAS and maternal feelings surrounding the infant's NAS display, and how NAS may affect the infant's capacity for feeding at the breast are likely to positively influence the mother's ability to initiate and sustain breastfeeding. Safe sleep is a particularly important topic, which should be reinforced at multiple points in the prenatal and postnatal periods.

## The Substance-Exposed Infant

The substance-exposed infant may present their own independent problems that impair their ability to feed at the breast, and additionally may compound maternal lactation deterrents. These may include preterm birth, low birth weight, and other medical conditions. Medical interventions, such as medications, intravenous lines, monitor wires, gavage feedings, and NICU environments may also impair an infant's ability to feed at the breast. Many substance-exposed newborns experience neurobehavioral dysregulation in the early neonatal period, which can be due to and potentiated by multiple substance exposures.

## Neonatal Abstinence Syndrome (NAS) and Lactation

There are many nonmedical strategies to help promote breastfeeding and help prevent NAS that are addressed in Chapter 14. Rooming in, swaddling, kangaroo care, and nonNICU treatment have been shown to be helpful in preventing/ameliorating NAS. NAS is a group of signs and neurobehaviors that occur in the infant after discontinuation of exposure to substances taken by the mother. While typically associated with opioid exposures, other substances, such as nicotine, benzodiazepines, and SSRIs may cause an independent abstinence or toxidrome phenomenon, or may augment an opioid-induced NAS. Regardless of the antecedents of the NAS display in the infant, factors related to this disorder can and often do impair breastfeeding. Infants affected by NAS may display problems with motor control, such that they are hypertonic and/or jittery with uncontrolled and/or jerky movements. These infants are frequently difficult to position on the breast and often display head thrashing when approaching a nipple. Suck/swallow incoordination, another feature of NAS, may impair the ability of the breastfed infant to take in enough calories to offset his increased expenditures due to motor control issues, particularly in the early postnatal period when only colostrum is available. Regulatory problems, or the imbalance between the autonomic, motor, state control and attentional/interactive subsystems [38, 39], are also a hallmark of NAS.

These subsystems interact with each other and the environment in a continuous fashion, such that an infant with NAS expending any additional effort in any one subsystem, i.e. motor control, may not have sufficient energy to achieve homeostasis and balance in the others, i.e. attentional/interactional subsystems. The inability of the NAS-affected infant who is exhibiting problems with regulation to achieve a quiet alert state which is necessary for breastfeeding can easily derail lactation in its early phases. Difficulties with state control, and tendency to be easily overstimulated, common features of infants with NAS, can also impair breastfeeding. These infants often go from sleep to an insulated crying state without reaching the quiet alert state that is necessary for feeding at the breast. Infants with NAS are often irritable and transmit poorly interpretable cues to their mothers, which may prompt the mother to soothe the infant with her breast if she interprets all crying as hunger. This can result in the infant at the breast for most or all of the day, never taking a full feeding and disrupting wake/sleep cycles. Medication for NAS, typically morphine or methadone, can also impair breastfeeding capabilities in infants who are sedated after medication, or overstimulated prior to medication to latch at the breast without medication. For infants that require prolonged hospitalization, prolonged separation may inhibit the mother's ability to pump breastmilk for her infant. These difficulties can be further compounded by a mother that experiences guilt, easy frustration, or poor tolerance for her inability to feed or soothe the infant. Lastly, infants who are breastfed tend to have shorter sleep/wake cycles, which can negatively affect their NAS scoring. It is prudent to adapt NAS scoring to the breastfed infant by disallowing increased NAS scores for physiologic sleep cycles that are less than 3 hours.

## Treating the Breastfeeding Infant of a Mother with an SUD

When considering lactation for the substance-exposed infant, a thorough understanding of their longitudinal health status, medications, environment, and NAS display is warranted, as these factors are likely to change and evolve with time. Understanding the infant's dyadic communication pattern and triggers for dysregulation or overstimulation requires careful observation of the infant with his mother during breastfeedings, routine cares, and other interactions. Evaluation of the infant's response to external stimuli, such as auditory, visual, or tactile stimuli will provide a mechanism to assess his triggers for dysregulatory behaviors that will impact breastfeeding. Similar assessment of the infant's response to internal stimuli, such as bowel movements or hunger, will allow interpretation of his capacity to cue his caregivers for necessary interventions. Promoting the mother's capacity for recognizing and interpreting signs of infant hunger, discomfort, fatigue, or dysregulation will assist her ability to provide contingent and sensitive responses. These responses can be learned and should be adaptable to the infant's changing condition over time. All infant crying is not hunger, and constant breastfeeding or using the maternal breast as a pacifier to soothe an irritable infant should be avoided, as in these cases the infant never receives a full feed and the maternal breast is never completely emptied, and it may additionally predispose the nipples to cracking/bleeding which may present risk for women with HCV infection.

Observation of the breastfeeding infant will allow the provider to assess factors that can impair lactation, such as factors related to NAS including hypertonicity, suck swallow incoordination or overstimulation, and simultaneously allow the modification of handling and/or the environment to overcome these difficulties (see Figure 15.1). It is important to note that the feeding capacity of some infants is affected by the timing of medication administration delivered coincident with each feeding. Some infants cannot be positioned on the breast without medication, some may require medication during or after a feed, or a split dose of medication delivered before and after a feed to be able to breastfeed successfully.

## The Provider, Institution and Environment, and the Lactating Woman with SUD

### The Provider

The typical obstetric or pediatric provider or lactation consultant is often not adequately prepared to treat the substance-exposed dyad, yet it is these providers that are more often than not expected to provide optimal

| Infant NAS sign | Breastfeeding intervention |
| --- | --- |
| **Motor and tone control problems**<br>Hypertonia<br>Jitteriness<br>Head thrashing<br>Arching | Avoid infant positioning on the breast in any position that promotes back arching or hypertonia; i.e. one infant arm behind the mother's back. Swaddle the infant to reduce tremors, bring arms and legs forward and curve the infant's body in a C position. Apply gentle pressure to the occiput if tolerated. |
| **State control/attentional problems/sensory sensitivity**<br>Poor behavioral state control (abrupt changes, difficulty in achieving states appropriate for feeding)<br>Sensory processing difficulties (sensory over or under responsivity) | Identify interactional and environmental interventions (i.e. avoiding eye contact, rocking, dim light, pacifier) that help the newborn to achieve a drowsy or quiet alert state to start the breastfeeding. Decrease any visual, auditory, tactile stimuli that may dysregulate the infant. When medication is needed avoid sedation if present by administering the medicine in the middle or after feeding; consider splitting the dose. |
| **Autonomic instability**<br>Fever<br>Tachypnea<br>GI disturbances (vomiting, loose stools, "gas") | Identify autonomic signs that may indicate sensory stress and avoid their external or internal triggers: (visual/auditory), tactile (blankets, pressure points, monitor wires), excessive gas due to limited burping. Swaddling; may need to restrict to extremities if fever present. Small frequent breastfeedings on demand, modifying the Finnegan score to reflect this intervention (i.e. do not score for sleeping less than 3 hours for breastfed infants who feed more frequently). |
| **Suck/swallow incoordination**<br>Formula loss at sides mouth | Chin support if helpful. Avoid gavage feedings, which will worsen other symptoms of NAS, when possible. Monitor infant weight. May require OT consultation. |

**Figure 15.1** NAS neurobehaviors and breastfeeding interventions

care to this high-risk population. Many do not have adequate training in, or understanding of substance use disorders and the myriad issues surrounding the substance-exposed dyad, and breastfeeding, deemed by many providers as a privilege to be earned for this group, is easily derailed in this circumstance. Hospital-based nurses in particular may undermine breastfeeding efforts [6]. Pejorative attitudes, whether overtly or covertly expressed, not infrequently lead to formula feeding even when breastmilk is available (i.e. "I do not know what is in this breastmilk and I am responsible for the care of this infant, therefore the infant will receive formula"), which can result in miscommunication and unhelpful confrontations with mothers. There often exists a dearth of available information necessary to develop appropriate interventions for the mother with SUD who expresses a desire to breastfeed. Women who are not engaged in prenatal care or SUD treatment or who have an active addiction are not appropriate candidates for lactation. Mothers with SUDs are often poor historians due to the multiple pressures to deny substance use in the perinatal period. Commonly used biologic toxicology screens (i.e. urine toxicology testing) only reflect recent substance use or misuse in most cases (exceptions are THC for with chronic use or benzodiazepines) and are of limited value. Negative results do not rule out an SUD, positive results do not quantify use, none are of use in detecting use early in pregnancy, and women with SUD who are in active addiction patterns can produce negative results by "rigging" their urine (i.e. providing someone else's urine) to avoid detection. Other screens, such as umbilical cord tissue and meconium, are being used more commonly today and reflect a longer period of exposure for the infant (i.e. back to the second trimester), but may not reflect periods of abstinence closer to delivery, which are particularly important to note in women in SUD treatment, and are not particularly sensitive in detecting lipophilic substances such as methamphetamines [40, 41]. Infants who are opioid-exposed are typically held for 4–5 days for observation for the development of NAS, and this period is useful in the establishment of lactation. However, when substance exposure is unrecognized, infants can be discharged as early as the second day of life, and for dyads at risk for failure of lactation, this period is inadequate to allow interventions that may benefit lactation, and increases the likelihood that an infant may have NAS after discharge which may be dangerous. All infants of mothers without prenatal care could benefit from social services and home visits for the assessment of the home environment, provision of necessary services such as transportation to infant checks and postpartum visits, and close observation of possible NAS symptom expression.

Guidelines for the purposes of encouraging/discouraging lactation are often unclear [42]; in general, breastfeeding for substance-exposed infants is generally encouraged by the AAP and ACOG under certain circumstances which may not be easy to discern [43, 44]. One consistent guideline is that any active illicit substance use/licit substance misuse patterns are not compatible with lactation; however, there is evidence that, for marijuana at least, providers are promoting lactation regardless of active use [45]. Providers often do not have time or institutional support to treat the dyad as opposed to their own (i.e. the obstetric or pediatric) patient, in which cases reimbursement for services may not be provided. Unclear legal risks of promoting breastfeeding in a woman with an SUD are a further concern, particularly for marijuana, which is now a legal substance in many areas. It may be legally ill-advised to promote breastfeeding in marijuana using mothers [46] because it is still a Category I controlled drug, illegal under federal law (despite state laws), and against CDC, AAP and ACOG guidelines. Perhaps more importantly, it may be a missed opportunity to provide treatment for an SUD or services to an at-risk infant by promoting breastfeeding in these dyads. However, it is difficult to assess when a woman undergoing SUD treatment for marijuana use should be allowed to breastfeed as urine toxicology can remain positive for weeks to months. Certainly, if there is active engagement with SUD treatment without evidence of active use, breastfeeding can still be encouraged.

## The Environment

The environment is also important to consider in the promotion of lactation in women with SUD [47]. A history of sexual abuse may make routine care of the lactating mother on a busy postpartum floor difficult. While there is increasing evidence that rooming in care may be optimal for the dyad [48] and may improve breastfeeding rates among substance-exposed dyads, it is not always possible if there are outstanding maternal or infant medical needs, maternal psychosocial concerns or limitations of the hospital. Visiting family or significant other concerns (i.e. "the baby may OD"), or mistrust of the mother to be able to provide nutrition for the infant in the face of previous poor health choices can derail even the most stolid breastfeeder. NICUs and newborn nurseries are often not ideal for substance-exposed newborns, and bright lights, loud noises, rough handling or physical accoutrement such as monitor wires, security devices, and rough linens can all potentiate NAS which in turn can exacerbate breastfeeding difficulties. Multiple and changing handlers, such as nurses, therapists, and physicians who may not be familiar with the plan for lactation can easily opt to provide formula for an infant they deem needs it in the absence of the mother, who may have important SUD treatment facility or social services requirements.

## Modifying the Provider Approach and the Environment to Support Lactation in Women with SUD

As both the mother and the infant should be thoroughly evaluated for optimal breastfeeding, so should the provider and the environment. Institutions should have clearly thought out guidelines for breastfeeding by women with SUD [47]. Each provider should have clear guidelines for encouraging/discouraging breastfeeding that are equitably applied and do not vary by substances used/misused or socioeconomic status of the mother. Formula should not be the default feeding for every substance-exposed infant, and it should not be offered or provided at the first sign of lactation difficulties, but should be provided in instances where maternal sobriety, engagement in SUD treatment or mental health stability is threatened; in these cases, gentle "permission" to formula feed should be given. While breastfeeding provides optimal nutrition, it is ultimately the mother's progress in or acceptance of SUD treatment and sobriety that are of paramount importance to the infant's health and development.

Health care provider attitudes and existing knowledge often need adjustment when treating women with SUD. A nonjudgmental, nonpunitive approach is crucial, as many women with SUD have had difficult experiences with medical care providers or institutions. At least a working knowledge of addictions and the understanding of addiction as a chronic relapsing disease that can respond to treatment is also important. Providers should beware of miscommunications that may derail breastfeeding, such as mixed messages from staff regarding the suitability for breastfeeding for each woman, or pejorative language (i.e. "methadone baby," "addicted infant," "your breastfeeding difficulties are your own fault").

The physical environment may also need to be modified. For infants with NAS, it is important to avoid suboptimal physical environments, i.e. the NICU, or

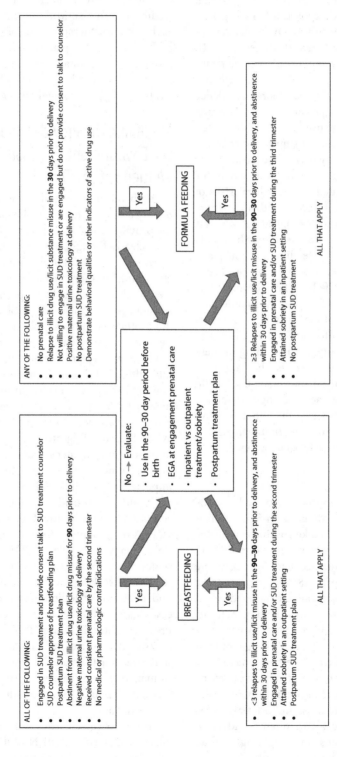

**Figure 15.2** Guidelines for the determination of breastfeeding candidacy for women with SUD

ALL OF THE FOLLOWING:
- Engaged in SUD treatment and provide consent talk to SUD treatment counselor
- SUD counselor approves of breastfeeding plan
- Postpartum SUD treatment plan
- Abstinent from illicit drug use/licit drug misuse for **90** days prior to delivery
- Negative maternal urine toxicology at delivery
- Received consistent prenatal care by the second trimester
- No medical or pharmacologic contraindications

No → Evaluate:
- Use in the 90–30 day period before birth
- EGA at engagement prenatal care
- Inpatient vs outpatient treatment/sobriety
- Postpartum treatment plan

ANY OF THE FOLLOWING:
- No prenatal care
- Relapse to illicit drug use/licit substance misuse in the **30** days prior to delivery
- Not willing to engage in SUD treatment or are engaged but do not provide consent to talk to counselor
- Positive maternal urine toxicology at delivery
- No postpartum SUD treatment
- Demonstrate behavioral qualities or other indicators of active drug use

BREASTFEEDING

FORMULA FEEDING

Yes

Yes

Yes

Yes

- <3 relapses to illicit use/licit misuse in the **90–30** days prior to delivery, and abstinence within 30 days prior to delivery
- Engaged in prenatal care and/or SUD treatment during the second trimester
- Attained sobriety in an outpatient setting
- Postpartum SUD treatment plan

ALL THAT APPLY

- ≥3 Relapses to illicit use/licit misuse in the **90–30** days prior to delivery, and abstinence within 30 days prior to delivery
- Engaged in prenatal care and/or SUD treatment during the third trimester
- Attained sobriety in an inpatient setting
- No postpartum SUD treatment

ALL THAT APPLY

suboptimal physical interventions, i.e. gavage feedings, when appropriate to do so. For women with sexual trauma histories, routine care in the perinatal period may need to be modified, including asking permission to touch the body, restricting nighttime care and male staff when necessary, and providing privacy while breastfeeding or pumping, or when exposing breasts or other body parts. Breast pumps should be available for women unable to get the infant comfortably on the breast, and should continue to be available to women whose infants remain hospitalized past the woman's hospital discharge. All women in SUD treatment receiving methadone or buprenorphine have an SUD treatment provider, who should provide useful maternal information given written permission from the mother to do so. Finally, and importantly, for any woman with an SUD who desires to breastfeed, the support of a lactation consultant familiar with NAS and maternal addictions is often a vital component to breastfeeding success.

There are multiple benefits to breastfeeding and breastmilk for both aspects of the substance-exposed dyad, and strategies to encourage lactation while overcoming often existent barriers [49] are methods of optimizing care for this vulnerable population of high-risk infants and women. Please see Figure 15.2 for suggested guidelines for the practitioner to evaluate the advisability of breastfeeding in most individual dyads.

# References

1. Mack K., Jones C., Paulozzi L. Vital signs: overdoses of prescription opioid pain relievers and other drugs among women – United States, 1999–2010. https://www.cdc.gov/mmwr/preview/mmwrhtml/mm6226a3.htm.

2. Patrick S. W., Davis M. M., Lehmann C. U., Cooper W. O. Increasing incidence and geographic distribution of neonatal abstinence syndrome: United States 2009 to 2012. *Journal of Perinatology: Official Journal of the California Perinatal Association.* 2015; 35(8):650–5. doi:10.1038/jp.2015.36.

3. Cirillo C., Francis K. Does breast milk affect neonatal abstinence syndrome severity, the need for pharmacologic therapy, and length of stay for infants of mothers on opioid maintenance therapy during pregnancy? *Advances in Neonatal Care.* 2016; 16(5):369–78.

4. Jansson L. M., Velez M. L., Harrow C. Methadone maintenance and lactation: a review of the literature and current management guidelines. *Journal of Human Lactation.* 2004; 20(1):62–71.

5. Kim P., Feldman R., Mayes L. C., et al. Breastfeeding, brain activation to own infant cry, and maternal sensitivity. *Journal of Child Psychology and Psychiatry.* 2011; 52(8):907–15.

6. Demirci J. R., Bogen D. L., Klionsky Y. Breast-feeding and methadone therapy: the maternal experience. *Substance Abuse.* 2014; 4:1–6.

7. Wachman E. M., Byun J., Philipp B. L. Breastfeeding rates among mothers of infants with neonatal abstinence syndrome. *Breastfeeding Medicine.* 2010; 5(4). doi: 10.1089=bfm.2009.0079.

8. CDC. Breastfeeding Report Card: United States, 2014. www.cdc.gov/breastfeeding/pdf/2014breastfeeding reportcard.pdf

9. Rutherford H., Williams S. K., Moy S., Mayes L. C., Johns J. M. Disruption of maternal parenting circuitry by addictive process: rewiring of reward and stress systems. *Frontiers in Psychiatry.* 2011 Jul 6; 2:37. doi: 10.3389/fpsyt.2011.00037.

10. DiSantis K. I., Collins B. N., McCoy A. C. Associations among breastfeeding, smoking relapse, and prenatal factors in a brief postpartum smoking intervention. *Acta obstetricia et gynecologica Scandinavica.* 2010; 89(4):582–6.

11. Frank D. A., Bauchner H., Zuckerman B. S., Fried L. Cocaine and marijuana use during pregnancy by women intending and not intending to breastfeed, Research and Professional Briefs. *Journal of the American Dietetic Association.* 1992; 2(92):215–17.

12. Substance Abuse and Mental Health Services Administration, Office of Applied Studies. *The NSDUH Report: Substance Use Among Women During Pregnancy and Following Childbirth.* Rockville, MD: Substance Abuse and Mental Health Services Administration; 2009. www.openminds.com/wp-content/uploads/indres/052109nsduhpregnancysu babuse.pdf. Accessed March 15, 2017.

13. Cone E., Bigelow G. E., Herrmann E. S., et al. Nonsmoker exposure to secondhand cannabis smoke. III. Oral fluid and blood drug concentrations and corresponding subjective effects. *Journal of Analytical Toxicology.* 2015; 1–13.

14. Winecker R. E., Goldberger B. A., Tebbetz I. R., et al. Detection of cocaine and its metabolites in breast milk. *Journal of Forensic Sciences.* 2001; 46(5): 1221–3.

15. Chasnoff I. J., Lewis D. E., Squires L. Cocaine intoxication in a breast-fed infant. *Pediatrics.* 1987; 80:836–8.

16. Chomchai C., Chomchai S., Kitsommart R. Transfer of methamphetamine (MA) into breast milk and urine of postpartum women who smoke MA tablets during pregnancy: implications for initiation of breastfeeding. *Journal of Human Lactation.* 2016; 32(2):333–9.

17. Bartu A., Dusci L. J., Ilett K. F. Transfer of methylamphetamine and amphetamine into breast milk following recreational use of methylamphetamine. *British Journal of Clinical Pharmacology.* 2009; 67(4):455–9.

18. Ariagno R., Karch S. B., Middleberg R., Stephens B. G., Valdes-Dapena M. Methamphetamine ingestion by a breast-feeding mother and her infant's death: People v Henderson. *JAMA.* 1995; 274:215.

19. Kaufman K. R., Petrucha R. A., Pitts F. N. Jr, Weekes M. E. PCP in amniotic fluid and breast milk: case report. *Journal of Clinical Psychiatry.* 1983 Jul; 44(7):269–70.

20. Mennella J. Alcohol's effect on lactation, 2012. http://pubs.niaaa.nih.gov/publications/arh25-3/230-234.htm. Accessed March 15, 2017.

21. Giglia R., Binns C. Alcohol and lactation: a systematic review. *Nutrition & Dietetics.* 2006; 63:103–16.

22. Kelly L. E., Poon S., Madadi P., Koren G. Neonatal benzodiazepines exposure during breastfeeding. *The Journal of Pediatrics.* 2012; 161:448–51.

23. Rubin E. T., Lee A., Ito S. When breastfeeding mothers need CNS-acting drugs. *Canadian Journal of Clinical Pharmacology.* 2004; 11:257–66.

24. Lam J., Kelly L., Ciszkowski C., et al. Central nervous system depression of neonates breastfed by mothers receiving oxycodone for postpartum analgesia. *Journal of Pediatrics.* 2012; 160:33–7.

25. Hendrickson R. G., McKeown N. J. Is maternal opioid use hazardous to breast-fed infants? *Clinical Toxicology (Philadelphia, PA).* 2012; 50(1):1–14.

26. United States Food and Drug Administration. www.fda.gov/Drugs/DrugSafety/ucm118113.htm. Accessed April 26, 2017.

27. ElSohly M. A. *Potency Monitoring Program Quarterly Report No. 123 – Reporting Period: 09/16/2013–12/15/2013.* Oxford: University of Mississippi, National Center for Natural Products Research, 2014.

28. Perez-Reyes M., Wall M. E. Presence of D9-tetrahydrocannabinol in human milk. *The New England Journal of Medicine.* 1982; 307:819–20.

29. Fernando-Ruiz J., Gomez M., Hernandez M., et al. Cannabinoids and gene expression during brain development. *Neurotoxicity Research.* 2004; 6: 389–401.

30. Liston J. Breastfeeding and the use of recreational drugs, alcohol, caffeine, nicotine and marijuana. *Breastfeeding Review.* 1998; 6:27–30.

31. Garry A., Rigourd V., Amirouche A., et al. Cannabis and breastfeeding. *Journal of Toxicology.* 2009; 596149 Epub 2009 Apr 29.

32. Kozhimannil K. B., Graves A. J., Levy R., Patrick S. W. Predictors of prescription opioid abuse among pregnant US women. *Women's Health Issues.* 2017; 27(3):308–15. doi: 10.1016/j.whi.2017.03.001.

33. Jansson L. M., Choo R., Velez M. L., et al. Methadone maintenance and breastfeeding in the neonatal period. *Pediatrics.* 2008; 121(1):106–14.

34. Jansson L. M., Spencer N., McConnell K., et al. Maternal buprenorphine maintenance and lactation. *Journal of Human Lactation.* 2016; 32(4):675–81.

35. Velez M. L., Montoya I. D., Jansson L. M., et al. Exposure to violence among substance-dependent pregnant women and their children. *Journal of Substance Abuse Treatment.* 2006; 30:31–8.

36. Kendall-Tackett K. Breastfeeding and the sexual abuse survivor. *Journal of Human Lactation.* 1998 Jun; 14(2):125–30.

37. Kendall-Tackett K., Cong Z., Hale T. W. Depression, sleep quality, and maternal well-being in postpartum women with a history of sexual assault: a comparison of breastfeeding, mixed-feeding, and formula-feeding mothers. *Breastfeeding Medicine.* 2013 Feb; 8(1): 16–22.

38. Als H. Toward a synactive theory of development: Promise for the assessment and support of infant individuality. *Infant Mental Health Journal.* 1982; 3(4):229–43.

39. Jansson L. M., Velez M. Neonatal abstinence syndrome. *Current Opinion in Pediatrics.* 2012; 24(2):252–8.

40. Derauf C., Katz A. R., Easa D. Agreement between maternal self-reported ethanol intake and tobacco use during pregnancy and meconium assays for fatty acid ethyl esters and cotinine. *American Journal of Epidemiology.* 2003; 158(7):705–9.

41. Wright T. E., Milam K. A., Rougee L., Tanaka M. D., Collier A. C. Agreement of umbilical cord drug and cotinine levels with maternal self-report of drug use and smoking during pregnancy. *Journal of Perinatology: Official Journal of the California Perinatal Association.* 2011; 31(5):324–9.

42. Reece-Stremtan S., Marinelli K. A. Academy of breastfeeding medicine. ABM clinical protocol #21: guidelines for breastfeeding and substance use or substance use disorders, revised. *Breastfeeding Medicine.* 2015; 10:135–41.

43. Section on Breastfeeding, American Academy of Pediatrics. Breastfeeding and the use of human milk. *Pediatrics.* 2012; 129(3):e827–41.

44. Committee on Health Care for Underserved Women and the American Society of Addiction Medicine. *Opioid Abuse, Dependence, and Addiction in Pregnancy.* ACOG Committee Opinion No. 524. 2012; 1–7.

45. Bergeria C. L., Heil S. H. Surveying lactation professionals regarding marijuana use and

breastfeeding. *Breastfeeding Medicine.* 2015; 10(7):377–80.

46. E Stanton, Esq. Vermont Oxford Network, 2014. Holmes A. V., Atwood E. C., Whalen B., et al. Rooming-in to treat neonatal abstinence syndrome: improved family-centered care at lower cost. *Pediatrics.* 2016 Jun;137(6). pii: e20152929. doi: 10.1542/peds.2015-2929.

47. Patrick S. W., Schumacher R. E., Horbar J. D., et al. Improving care for neonatal abstinence syndrome. *Pediatrics.* 2016; 137(5). doi: 10.1542/peds.2015-3835.

48. Holmes A. V., Atwood E. C., Whalen B., et al. Rooming-in to treat neonatal abstinence syndrome: improved family-centered care at lower cost. *Pediatrics.* 2016; 137(6). pii: e20152929.

49. Jansson L. M., Velez M. Lactation and the substance-exposed mother–infant dyad. *The Journal of Perinatal & Neonatal Nursing* 2015 Oct–Dec; 29(4):277–86.

# Index

Printed in the United States
by Baker & Taylor Publisher Services